CW00346093

Dr Chandra Patel is an internationall⟨
on the prevention and control of high ⟨
management of heart disease. For the l⟨
has worked as a General Practitioner in
interest in helping patients with heart ⟨
rather than being totally reliant on dru⟨
was also a member of the executive board of the South West
Thames Faculty of the Royal College of General Practitioners.
In 1980 she was awarded the British Heart Foundation
"Doctor" award and in 1981 the James Mackenzie Award for
her research in cardiovascular medicine. She is now Senior
Clinical Lecturer in the Department of Community Medicine,
University College London and Middlesex Hospital Medical
School. She has recently been made an Honorary Fellow of the
Society of Behavioral Medicine of the United States.

Dr Patel has written numerous articles for medical journals
on the prevention and management of hypertension and
coronary heart disease, principally through yoga, relaxation
and biofeedback.

THE BRITISH HOLISTIC MEDICAL ASSOCIATION

FIGHTING HEART DISEASE

Dr Chandra Patel
MB BS MD MRCGP

☐☐☐☐☐SERIES EDITOR☐☐☐☐☐
Dr Patrick C. Pietroni
MB BS FRCGP MRCP

LONDON • NEW YORK • SYDNEY • MOSCOW

Contents

To

HIRU
PANKAJ, MALINI, SMRUTI,
SANGEETA AND VIKRAM

Project editor Jemima Dunne

Art editor Philip Lord

Managing editor Daphne Razazan

First published in Great Britain in 1987 by
Dorling Kindersley Publishers Limited
9 Henrietta Street, London WC2E 8PS

www.dk.com

2 4 6 8 10 9 7 5 3 1

British Library Cataloguing in Publication Data

Patel, Chandra
Fighting heart disease.
1. Coronary heart disease – Prevention
I. Title
616.1'2305   RC685.C6

ISBN 0-86318-165-1 paperback
ISBN 0-86318-222-4 hardback

Printed in Hong Kong.

NOTE

Throughout this book the masculine pronoun 'he' is used when referring to the doctor or patient. This is for convenience and does not reflect a preference for either sex.

Preface

The British Holistic Medical Association was launched in 1983 to address a growing need amongst doctors, medical students, the practitioners of alternative, or complementary medicine and the public. This growing need was best expressed by H.R.H. the Prince of Wales when he spoke to the B.M.A. Conference. He suggested: *"Human nature is such that we are frequently prevented from seeing that what is taken for today's unorthodoxy is probably to be tomorrow's convention"*.

He went on to add: *"The whole imposing edifice of modern medicine, for all its breathtaking successes is like the celebrated Tower of Pisa, slightly off-balance"*.

"Balance" is a critical concept in "Holism". This new word is not synonymous with complementary or alternative and it must be stressed that the wholesale application of alternative medicine is not one of the aims of the British Holistic Medical Association. Nor is an unthinking and self-destructive criticism of orthodox medicine appropriate. Holism is about responding to the whole person in his or her environment. It involves actively encouraging a partnership role between doctor and patient and nowhere is this more needed than in heart disease.

Heart disease is one of the most prevalent forms of dis-ease found in our culture. We have seen the tremendous benefits that technological medicine has produced in this area. Valve replacements, intensive care and heart transplants have caught the public imagination. Yet for the vast majority of patients, these advances are of little relevance. The problems of high blood pressure, heart failure and vascular disease all require appropriate diagnostic procedures. They also require treatment which takes into account not just the disease but the person as well. This book, which is the first of a series, will lay the groundwork for the medicine of the future – a true marriage between the best of technological medicine and the most appropriate therapies for helping the person regain his or her physical, mental and spiritual well-being.

Dr Patrick C. Pietroni MB BS FRCGP MRCP
Senior Lecturer in General Practice
St. Mary's Hospital Medical School, London

Foreword

Most heart attacks and strokes need not occur, if only we could put into practice the knowledge gained through medical research and embodied in some simple preventive recommendations, set out clearly by the World Health Organization.

Three things have stood in our way. The first is the media-fostered belief that we can leave it to high-technology medicine and surgery; the second is a lack of public knowledge of what can be done, and why; and the third, and perhaps most fundamental, has been a slowness of individuals and the community to accept that they are responsible for their own health. Happily, in all three respects the situation has been improving rapidly: and whereas until recently this excellent book would have fallen on stony ground, it will now find many readers eager to become better informed of the facts and the possibilities.

As an experienced general practitioner, Dr. Chandra Patel has the facility to express a wealth of technical information in plain English. She has also won an international reputation for her research into stress and cardiovascular diseases. Surveys have repeatedly shown how concerned people are about the effects of stress on their health and happiness, and many will be glad to find here much practical wisdom on how to understand the stress in their lives and how to cope with it better.

Success in fighting heart disease will come from a cooperation between doctors and the public. The role of the doctors is to inform, encourage and support: this book does just that. The role for the public is to judge and to act.

Geoffrey Rose DM BSc FRCP FFCM
Professor of Epidemiology
London School of Hygiene and Tropical Medicine,
University of London

Introduction

A good ruler once called a wise man to him and asked "What is the most valuable thing a man can have? I wish to give my people the greatest gift in the world". The wise man answered, "It is not yours to give. Every living man already possesses the most valuable thing in the world – life."

Life is so mysterious that, although everyone knows what it is like to be alive, no one can explain exactly what life is. We all, though, appreciate the importance of health to the quality of our lives. Now that we understand something of how the body works, we are also learning about the conditions under which the body fails to work properly. It is not only physical states, but also social, psychological, and cultural factors which together affect our health. The heart is extremely sensitive to emotional and psychological changes, as well as to physiological states, and heart disease is often a result of physical and psychological misuse.

The heart disease epidemic

Increased understanding of the biological factors in health, as well as the tremendous technological advances in medicine, have allowed doctors to prevent and treat all kinds of disorders including those of the heart and the circulation much more effectively. Unfortunately, though, this century's great advances in medicine have been partially offset by a massive increase in the number of people suffering from degenerative heart disease. Many of the infections which took their toll on the lives of children and young adults – such as polio, smallpox, diphtheria, typhoid, cholera and tuberculosis – have been virtually eliminated from the Western world. But, strange as it may seem, once a person gets beyond young adulthood, his life expectancy is only marginally better now than it was at the turn of the century. Disorders of the heart and circulatory system are the leading causes of death and disability. They now kill some 350,000 men and women annually in Britain – more than all other causes combined.

High blood pressure, when the heart pumps blood through the circulatory system too forcefully, damages the blood vessels and strains the heart. This serious condition now affects as many as 20 per cent of the adult population. Coronary heart disease, when the blood vessels supplying nutrients to the heart muscle are damaged, now accounts for one-third of all deaths. Yet around the turn of this century both of these conditions were very rare.

Why have these potentially killer diseases become so common, and what can be done about them? Part of the answer to the first question may be that more people now reach adulthood and old age because of the reduction in premature deaths. The other more important fact is – quite simply – that there has been a genuine increase in these disorders. So what causes them? The answer to this is – equally simply – that our environments, our personal habits and our behaviour all appear to be jointly responsible. If we are to prevent these disorders, we need to understand them and learn how to change our behaviour, lifestyles and reactions to the pressures of our environments.

Importance of prevention

Conventional medicine, in which the patient plays a passive role while the doctor treats the disease with pills and surgery, has failed to reduce the death toll so far. Prevention coupled with early intervention, involving active participation from the patient, seems to be the only answer.

There is strong evidence to show that if you accept an active role in maintaining your own health, you are much more likely to succeed in controlling your blood pressure and in preventing a heart attack or a stroke. This book explains how to take care of your own health and helps you to avoid heart problems and, if you already have heart disease, it will explain what you can do to promote recovery.

Stress and heart attacks

I remember a cardiologist colleague telling me how he suffered a heart attack. His research into stress and heart disease was being impeded and delayed by bureaucratic demands. The more frustrated he became with the bureaucratic machine, the greater his vigour in struggling against any obstacles. He worked faster and harder, neglecting rest and relaxation, family life and social activities.

One day, while lecturing to his students on heart attacks and sudden death, irony played its hand and he suffered his own heart attack. Ideally placed to receive immediate treatment, he was rushed to a coronary care unit. He survived. He remains convinced that he had brought his heart attack upon himself. He had pushed himself too hard, he had reacted emotionally to a stressful situation, and he had driven himself relentlessly in his aim for perfection – as consultant, teacher, public speaker and researcher. He learnt his lesson the hard way, and this is what he said about it afterwards: "It is only by coming close to death yourself that you realize that something terribly important is happening to people who are under stress."

The moral of this story is that the interaction between mind and body can make you ill. Likewise, it can make you well – and keep you well: there is a great deal you can do to enhance your health and enjoy a full and active life.

The holistic approach

The idea of the body as a purely mechanical system is falling out of favour. Doctors as well as the non-medical public are now beginning to recognize the importance of the mind's influence over the body. The conventional mechanical approach to medicine, in which blood pressure, cholesterol level and the structure of the blood vessels are viewed in isolation from the whole person, is now regarded as too narrow. We must extend our horizon to look at the person whose well-being is threatened, if we are to find out what has gone wrong and why it has failed. We must find answers to questions such as: What is his relationship with his family, his work and society? Is he under pressure from frustration and conflicts? How does he react to those pressures? How does he treat his body? Are his attitudes, lifestyle and behaviour upsetting the balance of his body, mind and spirit?

Many of the problems discussed in this book can be cured, at least partially, by a healthy diet, sufficient exercise, and an appropriate lifestyle. Relaxation, the way we appraise problems and our attitude to our environment all form a crucial part of treatment for many heart problems. Learning techniques such as proper breathing, deep muscle relaxation and even meditation, can make an important difference to our physical health and to our mental well-being. Meditation not only allows our bodies to recuperate, strengthens us emotionally and enriches us spiritually, it also has considerable beneficial physical effects on the heart and circulatory system.

My own enlightenment

The story of how I became interested in this subject is rather a curious one. After receiving undergraduate training at the University of London, followed by various hospital posts interspersed with numerous postgraduate courses, I finally joined a general practice in 1969. Armed with considerable diagnostic experience, the ability to recall scores of biochemical tests, and an extensive knowledge of pharmacopoeia, I thought that general practice was going to be a walkover. I was trained to believe that, at the roots of any disease, there was always some molecular derangement, biochemical depletion or structural defect; it could therefore be put right by medications to correct the biochemical abnormalities, or by surgery to remove or replace the diseased part.

I soon found that my entire system of belief was in turmoil. If illness was merely a question of molecular derangement, why did some patients take three weeks to recover from flu, while others were up and about in only three days? What about all those myriad aches and pains about which nothing was written in the text books? How come we had not been able to determine the causes of high blood pressure in 95 per cent of all those who were afflicted with it, in spite of the enormous wealth of technology behind us? Why did so many people feel permanently tired when we were unable to find anything organic to account for it? People consulted me

with mental, emotional and spiritual problems which did not fit into any diagnostic category. Even when the problems were apparently physical, a barrage of tests and X-rays often proved to be normal.

I began to feel that, on a number of occasions, prescriptions did not serve any purpose other than to cover up for my own incompetence. The high expectations of my patients were matched only by my anxiety to prove my worth, but I lacked the necessary skill. It is all too easy to lose courage and become despondent, and I was no exception. I suffered a duodenal ulcer and many restless, sleepless nights.

My medical practice was in a state of crisis. But sometimes out of crisis comes inventiveness – and so it was for me. One day, I recognized, quite suddenly, the similarities between my problems and those of my patients: no matter what our individual roles, they were not being fulfilled. Human potential was being wasted and depleted of all its creative energy. I gradually began to realize that to stay physically healthy, we must develop skills to cope with the demands made on us, raise our self esteem and cultivate congenial relationships and spiritual well-being.

On the right track

In order to heal myself, I took to practising what I had learned in my early days – slow abdominal breathing, yoga exercise, deep physical relaxation and meditation. Not only did I begin to feel physically fit and mentally peaceful, but I was also able to concentrate on the problems facing me, both as a person and as a general practitioner, and I succeeded in finding solutions. Not surprisingly, I became a good listener; I lent my patients support and in turn I received support from them. We all sensed that we were, at last, on the right track, and solutions were in sight.

My energy level was three times as high as it had been before. I worked long hours, found time to discuss in detail with my patients what might be the cause of their problems so that they could gain insight into them, and taught them both physical and mental relaxation. Sometimes we worked together to devise ingenious schemes to manage life's everyday pressures. It was as if we were all growing up together and reaching a state of new-found maturity.

The results of this process were that, for many of my patients, sleep became more peaceful, coping with everyday stress became easier, their interpersonal relationships improved, aches and pains became fewer and less troublesome and, coincidentally, their blood pressure was reduced. I was aware that high blood pressure was a killer disease, and so this reduction was certainly beneficial.

East meets West

Some interesting developments were occurring in medicine at the same time. The idea of patients controlling their own physiological functions through the concept of "mind over matter" was spreading. In the East, this idea was not new. It occurred to me that if we could combine Eastern philosophy with Western technology, it might be possible to achieve better results than we could expect from either approach on its own. What follows in the book is a mixture of age old wisdom and the most up-to-date information on causes, consequences, prevention and treatment of high blood pressure, coronary heart disease and related disorders.

The aim of this book

This book is addressed mainly to people who have already fallen victim to heart disease, and to those who would like to reduce the risk of developing heart problems. It will give you a clearer understanding of how the heart and circulatory system work and what can go wrong. It will also explain the types of examinations and tests you are likely to undergo before a diagnosis can be reached, and describe the conventional treatments for common heart problems.

Most important of all, the self-help section in the latter part of the book outlines how it is possible for you to develop your own healing powers and achieve the best possible health. No single aspect of the self-help strategies can be considered in isolation, but together they constitute a powerful weapon against the twin scourges of coronary heart disease and high blood pressure. I sincerely hope that the knowledge and experience I am sharing with you in this book will not only reward you with a longer life, but that it will also improve the quality of your life. And that, as the wise man said, is the most valuable thing in the world.

Acknowledgments

I would like to thank all the patients who provided me with the opportunity to try out many self-help techniques that helped me crystallize my ideas and made it possible to share my knowledge with others. I would also like to thank the many nurses and colleagues who have helped me over the years with research studies, especially Professor Tom Pilkington, Professor Michael Marmot, Professor Geoffrey Rose and Barbara Hunt. I am deeply grateful to the numerous colleagues and authors, both here and abroad, whose ideas and discoveries I have plundered. Specific acknowledgments for materials used in the book are given on page 192.

1
The healthy heart

A healthy heart is essential for the proper functioning of the entire body. The organs and tissues cannot survive without an adequate supply of oxygen, nutrients and warmth, and if waste matter is not taken away from them to be expelled from the body. The circulatory system, comprising the heart, the blood vessels and the blood, is the body's transport system: blood carrying oxygen and nutrients or waste matter is pumped round the body by the heart along the various tubes known as blood vessels (see opposite).

What is the heart?

The heart is a powerful muscular bag consisting of two pumps side by side, which pump blood to all parts of the body. Its steady beating maintains the flow of blood through the body day and night, year after year, non-stop from birth until death.

The amount of work performed by the heart is equivalent to a human being lifting 6kg (14lb) of weight to a height of 1.5m (5ft) every minute. After making such an effort a few times, a human being would become exhausted, but the heart never does – which is just as well, because the body cannot function without a constant supply of blood. The circulation, or cardiovascular system (involving both heart and blood vessels), is therefore of paramount importance to the continuation of life.

THE COMPOSITION OF BLOOD

Blood consists of several different types of cell (sometimes known as corpuscles) – red cells, white cells and platelets – suspended in a clear fluid known as plasma. The total amount of blood in the body is about 5 litres (8 pints).

Red cells are the most numerous type of blood cell; they outnumber white cells by 600 or 700 to one. Their most important component is a red pigment called haemoglobin, which is made up of iron known as haem and a protein called globin. Haemoglobin is important because it can combine with oxygen

in order to take the oxygen from the lungs to the body tissues. It also combines with carbon dioxide, a waste product in breathing, picking it up in the tissues when it gives up its oxygen and carrying it back to the lungs. Sufficient iron in the diet is essential to the production of haemoglobin.

White cells protect the body from infection, both by attacking microbes and by producing antibodies to provide immunity from invading microbes. There are several types of white cell each with a slightly different function.

BLOOD CIRCULATION

The blood makes two separate circuits from and to the heart known as the systemic circulation and the pulmonary circulation. In the systemic circulation, bright red blood containing oxygen is pumped from the left side of the heart into the main blood vessel in the body, the aorta, then into a series of tubes called arteries. These divide into smaller and smaller arteries throughout the body to supply the organs and tissues with oxygen and nutrients and to pick up waste products such as carbon dioxide. After leaving the tissues blood flows into veins, which join up and eventually form two large veins, the superior and inferior vena cavae, before returning to the heart, this time to the right side.

In the pulmonary circulation, the oxygen-depleted — or "used" — blood, which is slightly blue or purplish in colour because it has given up some of its oxygen on its way round the body, is pumped to the lungs. Here it takes in fresh supplies of oxygen and expels carbon dioxide. The newly oxygenated blood then returns to the left side of the heart then out into the body.

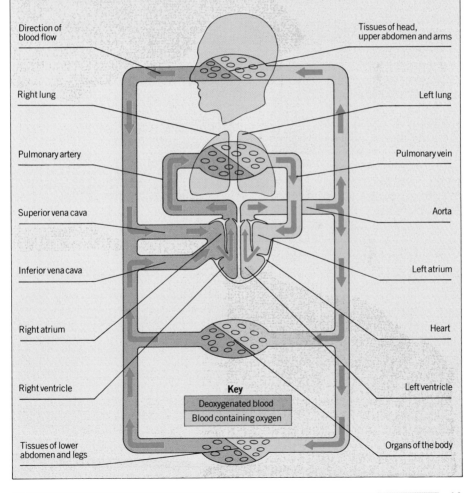

Direction of blood flow

Tissues of head, upper abdomen and arms

Right lung

Left lung

Pulmonary artery

Pulmonary vein

Superior vena cava

Aorta

Inferior vena cava

Left atrium

Right atrium

Heart

Right ventricle

Left ventricle

Key

Deoxygenated blood

Blood containing oxygen

Tissues of lower abdomen and legs

Organs of the body

Neutrophils and lymphocytes are two of the largest white cells.

Platelets are small blood cells which help plug an injury to a blood vessel in the first stage of clotting.

Plasma is a yellowish fluid in which the blood cells are suspended. It contains salts, proteins, antibodies and substances that aid clotting. Blood serum is the clear fluid left after all the various cells and proteins have been removed.

Blood cells

White blood cells

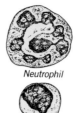

Neutrophil

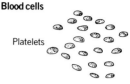

Platelets

Red blood cells

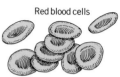

Lymphocyte

THE STRUCTURE OF THE HEART

The heart is a hollow, muscular organ slightly bigger than a clenched fist. It is situated just a little to the left of centre of the chest.

The walls of the heart are made of muscle which has a special contracting property. The heart is divided into two sides, each of which is further divided into an upper and a lower chamber – the atrium and the ventricle. The upper and lower chambers are linked by valves which open and close during heart beats to prevent a backflow of blood between beats. The valve on the left side has two cusps, or leaves, and is known as the mitral, or bicuspid, valve; the one on the right side has three leaves and is called the tricuspid valve.

Valves, known as semilunar valves, separate the ventricles from the blood vessels that carry blood away from the heart. The pulmonary valve separates the right ventricle from the pulmonary artery; the aortic valve separates the left ventricle from the aorta.

When the ventricles contract, the semilunar valves open, allowing blood to flow forwards. When the semilunar valves close, the tricuspid and mitral valves open and allow blood to flow through them into the relaxing ventricles. It is the closure of the different heart valves that produces the "lubb dubb" sounds which can be heard through a stethoscope.

Heart rate

In order for the heart to function efficiently as a pump, the heart muscles of the upper and lower compartments must contract in sequence. The rate at which the heart beats, or pumps, is controlled by its own natural "pacemaker". This consists of a group of specialized cells, call the sinoatrial node, situated in the wall of the right atrium. An electrical impulse is transmitted from the sinoatrial node to the

---

HEART FACTS

■ In an adult, the heart beats 60-72 times a minute at rest, accelerating to as many as 160-180 beats a minute during exercise, anxiety or fear.

■ It propels at least 5 litres (8 pints) of blood through a full circuit of the body every minute.

■ It beats some 100,000 times a day.

■ It pumps about 7,000 litres (1,500 gallons) of blood every day.

■ It could fill a 10km (6 mile) long goods train with blood in 60 years.

■ It generates enough power to drive a lorry round the world in four years.

BLOOD FLOW THROUGH THE HEART

"Used" blood returns to the heart through the veins which drain into two large channels called the superior and inferior venae cavae. Both of these drain into the right atrium, then through the tricuspid valve and into the right ventricle. On the next contraction, or heart beat, the muscular walls of the right ventricle push the blood through the pulmonary valve, along the pulmonary artery into the lungs. There the carbon dioxide is expelled and the blood is replenished with oxygen.

This oxygen-rich red blood then flows back through the pulmonary veins into the left atrium and through the mitral valve into the left ventricle. At the next heart beat, the left ventricle contracts, pushing the blood through the aortic valve and into the aorta.

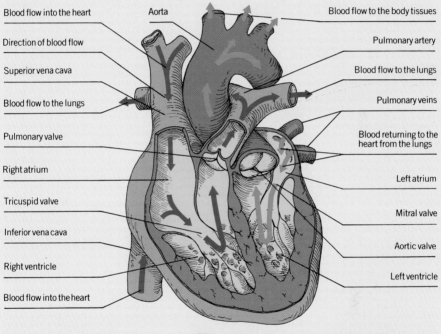

Blood flow into the heart

Aorta

Blood flow to the body tissues

Direction of blood flow

Pulmonary artery

Superior vena cava

Blood flow to the lungs

Blood flow to the lungs

Pulmonary veins

Pulmonary valve

Blood returning to the heart from the lungs

Right atrium

Left atrium

Tricuspid valve

Mitral valve

Inferior vena cava

Aortic valve

Right ventricle

Left ventricle

Blood flow into the heart

How the heart valves work
When the heart beats, the muscle contracts and forces blood through the heart (see overleaf). During contraction, the mitral and tricuspid valves close and the force of the blood flow pushes the pulmonary and aortic valves open. Between the contractions, the muscle relaxes, the pulmonary and aortic valves close and blood flows into the lower chambers pushing the other valves open.

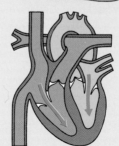

Atria contracting
Tricuspid and mitral valves open; pulmonary and aortic valves closed.

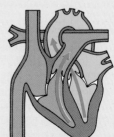

Ventricles contracting
Pulmonary and aortic valves open; tricuspid and mitral valves closed.

two atria, causing them to contract simultaneously. The electrical current then passes through to the walls of the ventricles, causing them, in turn, to contract simultaneously. The period of contraction is known as the systole. This is then followed by a short period of relaxation – about 0.4 seconds – known as the diastole, before the next impulse. The sinoatrial node produces between 60 and 72 of these impulses every minute when the heart is at rest. The production of these impulses is partially controlled by a part of the nervous system known as the involuntary, or autonomic, nervous system, which works without voluntary control.

It is this built-in electrical system that produces the rhythmic contractions of the heart muscles known as heart beats.

The electrical pathways
The electrical impulse is initiated in the sinoatrial node and passes into the walls of the atria, causing both chambers to contract. It then passes along fixed pathways to the atrio-ventricular node, into the walls of the left and right ventricles, causing the ventricles to contract.

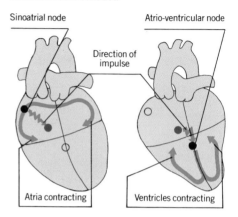

Sinoatrial node

Atrio-ventricular node

Direction of impulse

Atria contracting

Ventricles contracting

BLOOD VESSELS

Blood flows through a series of tubes, called blood vessels. These lead to and from the heart and carry blood to all parts of the body. There are approximately 96,000km (60,000 miles) of blood vessels in the body, of three main types: arteries, capillaries and veins.

Arteries
These are thick-walled blood vessels which carry blood away from the heart, either to the lungs or the rest of the body. The blood is forced along the arteries under such high pressure from the heart that the artery walls need to be strong and elastic. They expand with a surge of blood every time the heart beats, and this can be felt as a pulsation (see page 19). The arterial walls are made up of four layers: a membranous, smooth inner lining of cells; a layer of elastic tissue; a muscular wall; and a fibrous outer coating.

The arteries nearest to the heart are the largest, rather like motorways that lead away from a large city. The smaller arteries branch further into arterioles, like primary and secondary routes.

Capillaries
Arterioles divide and subdivide, like minor roads and footpaths, into a network of tiny, hair-like, thin-walled blood vessels called capillaries, from the Latin word *capillus*, meaning hair. These carry blood to every tissue of the body. Their thin walls allow the easy passage of oxygen and other nutrients in the blood to the body tissues, at the same time waste products pass from the tissues into the blood for their return journey to the heart.

Veins
The capillaries join up to form small venules and veins, which carry impure,

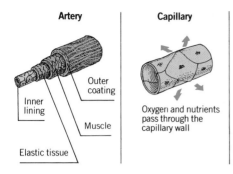

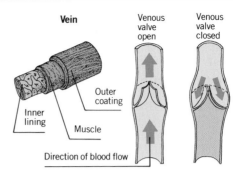

Artery	Capillary	Vein	Venous valve open	Venous valve closed

Artery: Inner lining, Outer coating, Muscle, Elastic tissue

Capillary: Oxygen and nutrients pass through the capillary wall

Vein: Inner lining, Outer coating, Muscle

Direction of blood flow

oxygen-depleted blood back to the heart. Since the blood in the veins is under much lower pressure than that in the arteries, the walls of the veins are thinner, less muscular and less elastic.

Veins are composed of three layers: a smooth, membranous lining; a thin layer of muscle; and an outer fibrous coating. They also have special valves at intervals which ensure that the blood flows in the right direction, towards the heart. Contraction and relaxation of the muscles during exercise squeezes the veins and helps to push the blood along.

BLOOD SUPPLY TO THE HEART

The heart, like any other organ, needs nutrition and this is supplied, via the coronary arteries, by a constant supply of blood, rich in oxygen and nutrients. The circulation in these arteries is therefore of the utmost importance.

There are two main coronary arteries, right and left, which branch off the main artery of the body, the aorta, very near its junction with the left ventricle, and encircle the heart like a crown – hence the word coronary, from the Latin word *corona*, meaning crown. The main arteries send out large branches, which cross over the surface of the heart, dividing and subdividing into smaller tributaries, which penetrate deep into the heart muscle to provide a constant and rich source of fresh blood.

The left coronary artery is the larger of the two coronary arteries. However, this artery quickly divides into two branches, which explains why doctors usually refer to three main coronary arteries: the right coronary artery; the left circumflex artery; and the left anterior descending artery, the last two being branches of the left main coronary artery. The right artery circles round the right side and goes to the back of the heart. The two left branches supply the front and left side of the heart.

Small blood vessels, known as collaterals, connect tributaries of the main coronary arteries. If a blockage occurs in one of the tributaries, it is likely that blood will still reach parts below the blockage because of these vascular links.

Coronary arteries

Aorta

Left coronary artery

Left circumflex

Right coronary artery

Left anterior descending artery

BLOOD PRESSURE

The blood is pumped under pressure from the heart through the blood vessels. Blood pressure is the force that is exerted against the walls of the blood vessels by the blood flowing through them. Or, in other words, blood pressure is the force that is required to circulate the blood round the body.

Pressure is highest in the arteries and arterioles, which conduct the blood from the heart to the rest of the body. It drops quite sharply in the capillaries, to allow nutrients and oxygen to pass from the blood into the body tissues. And it is lower still in the veins, which return impure blood to the heart. Unless you are specifically told otherwise by your doctor, blood pressure refers to the pressure in the arteries.

Systolic and diastolic pressure

The heart is not a continuous pump; it beats and then relaxes. Each heart beat produces a pressure wave, the peak of which occurs at the moment of contraction (systole), when the blood is pumped from the heart into the arteries. This is called the *systolic* pressure. The trough, or lowest point, occurs when the heart is relaxed during the interval between contractions (diastole), when the heart chambers are refilling. This is called the *diastolic* pressure.

Blood pressure is not a fixed quantity but varies considerably with everyday activities. It is dependent on two principal factors: the amount of blood expelled by the heart every minute, known as the cardiac output; and the degree of resistance, or calibre, of the arteries through which the blood flows, known as the peripheral resistance. Just as the pressure in a garden hose will increase when you turn the tap on more fully or constrict the opening of the hose, so blood pressure will increase if more blood is allowed to pass through the blood vessels, or if the blood vessels constrict for any reason.

The amount of blood passing through the heart is increased when the heart beats faster, pumping the same amount of blood with each stroke; or when a greater volume of blood flows out with each stroke, although the actual number of beats per minute remains the same. During the course of an ordinary day, blood pressure changes constantly: strenuous exercise or sudden stress makes it rise; a quiet rest makes it fall.

How blood pressure is regulated

Blood pressure is constantly changing in response to the day's stresses and exertions, and is controlled by a complex system of hormone release and built-in reflexes. One of these reflexes is achieved through special pressure-sensing cells, known as baroreceptors, which are scattered throughout the arteries and are capable of detecting the smallest changes in blood pressure. The most important baroreceptors are those in the walls of the aorta, the artery that carries blood away from the heart, and the two large arteries in the neck, the carotid arteries.

These cells function in a similar way to a thermostat in a central heating system. When the desired room temperature is set at a particular level in the thermostat, the thermostat attempts to maintain that level. Similarly, the baroreceptors are preset to a narrow range of blood pressure.

When the blood pressure rises above or falls below this range, the baroreceptors attempt to bring it back to within the preset range by initiating changes in the performance of the heart and in the calibre of the arteries. Thus when blood pressure is increased in the arteries, the baroreceptors send nerve signals to the brain. In response, the brain sends messages to the arteries, causing them to dilate, and to the heart, causing it to slow down, so allowing the blood pressure to fall. Alternatively, if the blood pressure falls – when you faint, for example – the opposite occurs: the arteries constrict and the heart quickens to restore pressure to normal.

POSITION OF THE BLOOD VESSELS

This diagram helps to illustrate how the circulatory system fits together in the body. Blood vessels carry blood to and from all parts of the body. Every time the heart beats, a wave of pressure passes along the arteries. These pulsations can be felt anywhere an artery is close to the surface of the body and are strongest in the large arteries. The most common places where they are felt are on the carotid artery in the neck, the radial artery at the wrist and the femoral artery in the groin.

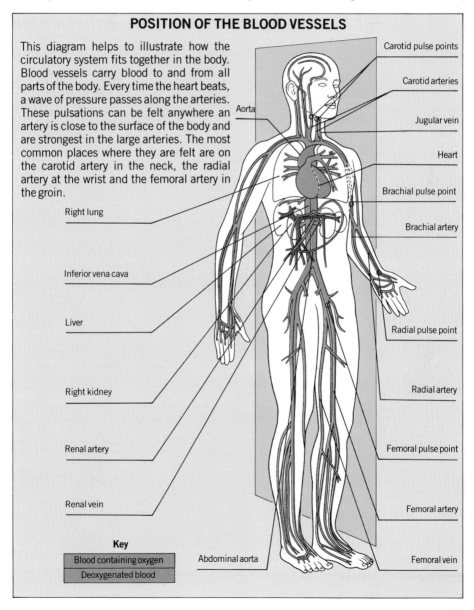

Carotid pulse points

Carotid arteries

Aorta

Jugular vein

Heart

Brachial pulse point

Brachial artery

Right lung

Inferior vena cava

Liver

Radial pulse point

Right kidney

Radial artery

Renal artery

Femoral pulse point

Renal vein

Femoral artery

Key

Blood containing oxygen

Deoxygenated blood

Abdominal aorta

Femoral vein

2
What can go wrong

Most of the time, the heart functions very well – particularly in view of the amount of work it does. We are, however, demanding more and more from our heart and our blood vessels – not perhaps directly but indirectly, through the amount we eat, drink and smoke, the pace of life and the risks to which we are exposed in the environment. It is hardly surprising, then, that things sometimes go wrong.

The chart below is intended as a quick guide to the problems that can occur. The term environment at the top of the chart means both the external environment and the internal one that exists within the body, mind and spirit.

Although we cannot always be sure precisely what causes each of the conditions listed, it is generally accepted that there is an interaction between hereditary and environmental factors.

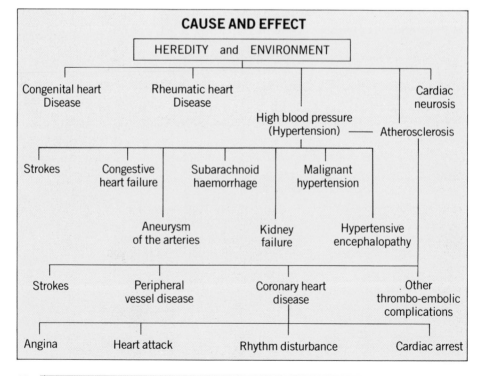

CAUSE AND EFFECT

HEREDITY and ENVIRONMENT

Congenital heart Disease

Rheumatic heart Disease

High blood pressure (Hypertension) —— Atherosclerosis

Cardiac neurosis

Strokes

Congestive heart failure

Subarachnoid haemorrhage

Malignant hypertension

Aneurysm of the arteries

Kidney failure

Hypertensive encephalopathy

Strokes

Peripheral vessel disease

Coronary heart disease

Other thrombo-embolic complications

Angina

Heart attack

Rhythm disturbance

Cardiac arrest

POSSIBLE DISORDERS

What follows is a description of each of the disorders mentioned on the flow-chart opposite. Their order follows the chart and does not bear any specific relationship to the incidence of the problem. Some of the rarer conditions are not described in any more detail in the rest of the book, but the more common problems, such as atherosclerosis, angina, high blood pressure and heart attacks are dealt with more fully in their own chapters later in the book.

Congenital heart disease

This is caused by heart malformations that are present from birth. Some of the deformities are so minor that they can be missed unless looked for. Others, such as the transposition of the great vessels, the aorta and the pulmonary arteries, or the presence of only one ventricle, are more obvious. In most crippling deformities, the deoxygenated, or "used", blood bypasses the lungs and continues to circulate around the body; this causes the characteristic colour of so-called "blue" babies.

Causes are not always clear, but certain factors during pregnancy, such as German measles, some drugs and even vitamin deficiency, have all been implicated. Some heart disorders run in families. Down's syndrome babies are more likely to have malformed hearts.

Those babies with congenital heart disease who do not have a blueness to their skin can be recognized by breathlessness on feeding because they find it difficult to suck; as such children grow older, they suffer from breathlessness

CONGENITAL DEFECTS

Illustrated below are two of the more common congenital defects. Ventricular septal defect, or hole in the heart, is a hole in the wall, or septum, between the two lower chambers of the heart. In about 25 per cent of these cases the hole will close; if the hole is large, surgery may be required.

The second defect occurs when the fetal circulatory system does not make the changes necessary for the baby to breathe on its own immediately after birth. Before birth, the fetus obtains oxygen from its mother via the placenta. To do this, the fetal heart has two bypasses, one of which, the ductus arteriosus, channels deoxygenated blood from the heart to the placenta to be oxygenated in the mother's lungs. This normally closes when the baby starts to breathe, but occasionally, this does not happen. If detected early, it can be corrected with drugs; otherwise surgery may be necessary.

Hole in the heart

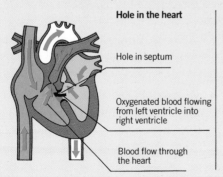

Hole in septum

Oxygenated blood flowing from left ventricle into right ventricle

Blood flow through the heart

Patent ductus arteriosus

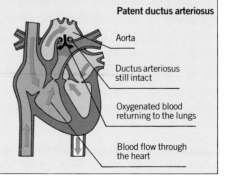

Aorta

Ductus arteriosus still intact

Oxygenated blood returning to the lungs

Blood flow through the heart

DAMAGE CAUSED BY RHEUMATIC FEVER

The extent of the damage to the heart caused by rheumatic fever is generally proportional to the number of attacks a person has.

Rheumatic fever can cause inflammation of the heart lining (endocarditis), or, rarely, of the heart covering (pericarditis) and the heart muscle itself (myocarditis).

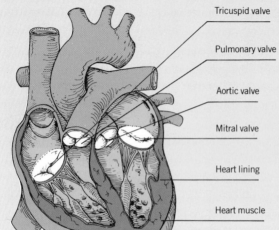

Tricuspid valve

Pulmonary valve

Aortic valve

Mitral valve

Heart lining

Heart muscle

Heart covering

Scarring of the valves
Damage to the valves caused by rheumatic fever can result in stenosis, or narrowing, of the valves, preventing them from opening properly, or incompetence, when the valve does not close properly, thus allowing back flow of blood.

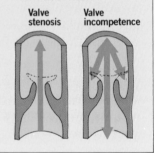

| Valve stenosis | Valve incompetence |

on exertion. Most heart defects can be corrected with surgery; fortunately, serious defects are uncommon.

Rheumatic heart disease

Rheumatic fever is not in itself a heart disease. About 60 per cent of all cases of rheumatic fever do, however, affect the heart. It tends to run in families and chiefly affects children between five and 15 years of age.

The fever is triggered by a throat infection caused by the streptococcal bacteria. The majority of sore throats nowadays are viral, and not all streptococcal infections lead to rheumatic fever, but if your child has a sore throat or feverish illness two to three weeks after a previous sore throat, consult your doctor.

In addition to fever, joint pains and in some cases, a sore throat, rheumatic fever can cause inflammation of various areas of the heart.

Once you have had rheumatic fever, you are prone to further attacks and, if it is not treated early, it can eventually lead to scarring of one or more of the heart valves in later life. In serious cases, surgery can be carried out to repair or replace damaged valves.

High blood pressure

If the force with which the blood flows in the circulation is much greater than normal, it is called high blood pressure, also known as hypertension. This puts the entire circulatory system, including the heart and blood vessels, under considerable strain. If high blood pressure persists for a number of years, it can lead to several complications. High blood pressure is described in more detail in Chapter 7.

Atheroma in the arteries
Fatty deposits called atheroma build up along the artery walls, reducing their diameter and elasticity; it is sometimes known as hardening of the arteries.

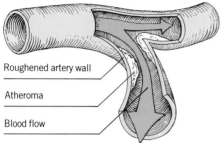

Roughened artery wall

Atheroma

Blood flow

Atherosclerosis

This is the process of silting up of arteries by deposits of fatty material called atheroma. The exact cause is not known but various risk factors increase the chances of atherosclerosis. The chief ones are a family history of this condition, age, cigarette smoking, a fatty diet, high blood pressure, obesity, lack of exercise and stress.

Atherosclerosis can affect any artery in the body. The possible consequences are angina, heart attack, stroke, kidney damage or peripheral vessel disease (ranging from cramps in the leg muscles to gangrene in an arm or leg). Atherosclerosis can largely be prevented. It is described fully in Chapter 6.

Cardiac neurosis

Not all chest pains are due to angina, (see page 27) or a heart attack (see page 27): there can be psychosomatic causes. Anxiety causes tension and, if it is not expressed in words or actions, the pent-up emotions express themselves as symptoms relating to any system in the body. When the heart is affected, it is known as neurocirculatory asthenia or psychosomatic heart disease.

The heart has long been regarded as the seat of emotion, so it is hardly surprising that anxiety and tension often have cardiovascular manifestations. The most common symptoms of this are palpitations, breathlessness and sharp stabbing pains in the region of the heart (often known as left submammary pain because the pain is below the left breast or nipple), associated with weakness, fatigue, shakiness or sweating. The symptoms can range from minor discomfort to complete invalidism.

The case history below is a good example of cardiac neurosis, although it should be remembered that not every case of non-specific chest pain is as extreme as this. Sometimes, a person is not even aware of any out-of-the ordinary stress. It is at a subconscious level but it affects his breathing and the way he feels and behaves. People with cardiac neurosis often breathe shallowly, using only the upper part of the chest.

A doctor is able to distinguish between angina (see page 27) and the pains of psychosomatic heart disease. In most cases, reassurance and simple psychotherapy are adequate. Exercise,

---

CASE HISTORY

Barry was 33 years old when he first complained of stabbing chest pains and palpitations. The symptoms usually started in the evening when he was resting. He had clammy hands and perspired profusely in his armpits. He was fairly fit and could climb several flights of stairs without experiencing any symptoms. A full medical examination revealed no abnormality and I was able to reassure Barry about the health of his heart.

Further probing revealed that he had had a vasectomy two years ago at a private clinic – a fact that he had kept secret from his wife, who was now pregnant. He continued to have minor symptoms, on and off, until his wife had the baby, after which he decided to confront her. They parted, and his symptoms did not return.

learning to breathe properly and relaxation will all help to clear up this condition (see Chapters 12 and 13).

Stroke

This is an interruption in the supply of blood to part of the brain which can lead to impaired function in the areas of the body controlled by that part of the brain. It can happen if a blood vessel in the brain bursts (cerebral haemorrhage), or is blocked by a blood clot (cerebral infarction). There are two types of cerebral infarction: thrombosis, when blood coagulates and blocks a cerebral artery, and embolism, when a blood clot elsewhere in the body is released into the blood stream and wedges in a cerebral artery.

Transient ischaemic attacks (TIA) are a form of mini stroke that result in slight sensory disturbance and/or muscle weakness lasting only a few minutes, and the patient always recovers completely within 24 hours.

Severe strokes may lead to unconsciousness, partial paralysis of one side of the body, speech problems, loss of memory, visual disturbances, and behavioural changes. Most patients will recover at least partially with a careful rehabilitation programme.

Congestive heart failure

Despite its name, heart failure is not an immediately life-threatening condition. It simply means that the heart cannot pump with enough force to continue efficient circulation. This may occur, for example, when the heart has to continue pumping blood into a hypertensive circulatory system. The heart eventually gets exhausted and blood does not flow through. This can result in a build-up of blood in the lungs, which in turn allows the fluid part of the blood, the plasma, to leak into the lungs, causing congested lungs and shortness of breath. It also causes fluid retention, usually resulting in swollen ankles. The heart muscle can also be weakened by infection, some degenerative changes (though the specific cause is not always known) or by a heart attack (see page 27).

Aneurysm

An aneurysm is a localized dilation, or bulging, in an artery. Aneurysms can occur anywhere, but they are most common and most troublesome when they are in a cerebral artery (see subarachnoid haemorrhage, opposite) or in the aorta. Atherosclerosis (see page 23 and Chapter 6) and high blood pressure (see page 22 and Chapter 7) may both cause a portion of the muscular layer of the artery wall to degenerate, allowing the lining to balloon out at the point of weakness. Other causes of aneurysm are congenital weakness in the artery wall and, rarely, arterial inflammation.

An aneurysm can create problems if a blood clot develops inside it, if it bursts, causing internal bleeding, or if it presses

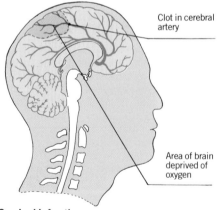

Clot in cerebral artery

Area of brain deprived of oxygen

Cerebral infarction
This is a blockage by a blood clot, of one of the arteries supplying blood to the brain. It results in the part of the brain supplied by that blood vessel being starved of oxygen.

ANEURYSMS

These may develop where there is a weakness in the artery wall. In one type the pressure of the circulating blood causes that part of the wall to bulge. Another type of aneurysm causes the inner and outer layers of an artery to split apart and blood to collect in between, causing the same balloon effect. Sometimes, a second split develops, which allows the blood clot back into the circulatory system.

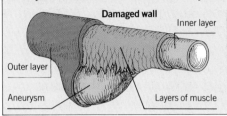

Damaged wall
Inner layer
Outer layer
Aneurysm
Layers of muscle

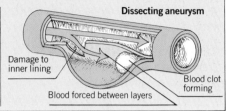

Dissecting aneurysm
Damage to inner lining
Blood clot forming
Blood forced between layers

on neighbouring organs, nerves or blood vessels. An aneurysm of the aorta is likely to cause turbulence in the flow of blood, which can, in turn, result in the formation of a clot. A piece of this blood clot may break away and lodge in any organ, interrupting its blood supply and causing damage to that organ. If the aneurysm is near the origin of the aorta, it may distort the aortic valve, thus making it incompetent – which means it does not close properly.

The best way to prevent an aneurysm is to guard against atherosclerosis (see page 23) and to keep your blood pressure under control. If, however, you develop a sensation of pressure or an inexplicable lump anywhere on the body, but especially on the abdomen, and particularly if it throbs, see your doctor as soon as possible as this could indicate an aneurysm. You will probably have a simple X-ray (see page 36) and an ultrasound scan. Then, if necessary, the doctor will arrange for a special X-ray called an arteriograph to be taken, to help identify the exact location and extent of the problem.

If an aneurysm has already occurred, it cannot be reversed but it can some-times be prevented from getting any bigger by a reduction in blood pressure.

It can also sometimes be surgically re-moved, and an artificial graft inserted.

Subarachnoid haemorrhage

Small aneurysms in the brain are called berry aneurysms. They are generally symptomless, but sometimes, an aneurysm causes symptoms, such as numbness, pins and needles, muscular weakness or headaches, in which case diagnosis can be made by a special brain X-ray called a CT Scan. Occasionally, one of the berry aneurysms bursts; this is especially likely if blood pressure is high. A sudden severe headache is felt at the back of the head and the person may become unconscious. This is called subarachnoid haemorrhage, because the blood collects in the space beneath the arachnoid membrane covering the brain. It is the most common cause of brain haemorrhage in younger people. A berry aneurysm can be surgically removed. Control of high blood pressure reduces the chances of one bursting.

Kidney failure

Amongst many other causes, long-standing high blood pressure can cause chronic kidney failure, also known as renal failure. We could in fact live quite happily with half a kidney but, because we have two, we have been endowed with such a large reserve that it takes many years of uncontrolled high blood pressure or other kidney disease before any signs of kidney failure come to the fore. Unfortunately, damaged kidneys are capable of raising blood pressure further, thus establishing a vicious circle. When kidneys are severely damaged, they are unable to carry out their function, which is to conserve water and some salts and to eliminate waste products and other salts.

If you find yourself passing abnormally large amounts of urine and also perhaps having to get up at night to pass urine, or have frequent headaches, breathlessness or an intensely itchy skin, you should consult your doctor. If you are also found to have high blood pressure, urine and blood tests are likely to be carried out and the doctor may refer you to a hospital for a special kidney X-ray called an intravenous pyelogram, or IVP for short. It may not be possible to revive the part of the kidney tissue that has already been destroyed, but it is possible to slow down its degeneration by treatment and diet under close medical supervision.

Malignant hypertension

This is the most serious form of high blood pressure, which can develop and progress very quickly, causing damage to the walls of the small arteries and arterioles. This damage can set such a tremendous inflammatory reaction in motion that sometimes these tiny vessels become completely clogged, shutting down the blood flow in them.

Since the kidneys are particularly rich in arterioles – they contain around a quarter of a million – damage to the kidneys is a hallmark of malignant hypertension. In turn, damaged kidneys can further raise blood pressure.

Other vital organs that can be affected by malignant hypertension are the brain and eyes.

Although high blood pressure on its own does not usually cause symptoms, malignant hypertension can cause headaches, giddiness and a general feeling of ill health. The safest thing is to go to your doctor, have your blood pressure measured, and let your doctor examine you (see Chapter 7).

Hypertensive encephalopathy

This term is used when the brain is affected by high blood pressure, usually of the malignant variety. It occurs only very rarely nowadays, because both the public and the medical profession are aware of the importance of measuring and controlling blood pressure.

It is due to a severe reduction in blood supply to the brain because of widespread damage to small blood vessels, as opposed to a stroke in which a major blood vessel becomes blocked. Attacks are heralded by severe headaches, nausea, vomiting or drowsiness, and there may be transient disturbance of the vision or speech, a feeling of disorientation, fits or unconsciousness.

Hypertensive encephalopathy is a medical emergency in which blood pressure has to be brought down from its dizzy heights, first with injections and then with drugs given by mouth. Recovery is usually complete, however, without any loss of function. Treatment usually has to be continued for the rest of the patient's life.

Peripheral vessel disease

Sometimes known as leg vessel disease, the medical term for this condition is intermittent claudication (from the Latin meaning limping or lameness). It is caused by atheroma building up in the arteries of the legs.

Leg vessel disease is particularly common in young active people who smoke. Initially there are no symptoms, but as the arteries become progressively narrower, pain occurs in the person's calf muscles and, less frequently, in the thigh and buttock muscles, on the affected side while walking. Occasionally, both legs are affected simultaneously. The distance that the person can walk before experiencing pain becomes shorter and shorter as the disease progresses – it may be no more than 50–100m (50–100yd) if the arteries are severely narrowed. The pain always comes on during exertion and disappears on standing still or resting. It is described variously as a dull ache, a vice-like squeezing pain, or cramp. It is caused by an inadequate supply of blood to the muscles during exercise, when they need more oxygen and fuel.

If you have this condition, the most important thing is to stop smoking. Drugs are available which are supposed either to dilate the arteries or to thin, or reduce the viscosity of, the blood, so allowing it to flow more easily. However, their effect is very limited because the drugs cannot actually stop the progression of the disease. It is more important to adopt self-help measures (see pages 124 to 186). Sometimes surgical treatment, in which an artificial graft is inserted to bypass the block, may restore the blood supply and cure the pain.

When they are severely narrowed, blood vessels may easily become completely blocked by a blood clot and the blood supply is cut off. Unless the vessel is large and can be bypassed by surgery, gangrene will result, the only treatment then being amputation.

Coronary heart disease

Also called coronary atherosclerosis, coronary artery disease or ischaemic heart disease, coronary heart disease is an umbrella term which refers to the narrowing of the coronary arteries by a build-up of atheroma and the consequences thereof, the main ones being angina and heart attack (see below and page 28). Often there are no symptoms of coronary heart disease, especially in the early stages. Sometimes a few of the linking blood vessels between the branches of the right and left coronary arteries (collaterals) enlarge to allow blood to bypass the narrowed vessels, in response to physical or nervous stress when the heart muscle needs an increased supply of blood.

However, if the blood supply to the heart muscle becomes inadequate during increased demands, angina pain develops. And if coronary heart disease continues untreated and the arteries become increasingly blocked, the blood supply to the heart may be reduced to such an extent that there is a risk of a heart attack (see Chapter 9).

Angina

Sometimes referred to as angina pectoris, this is not a disease in itself but a symptom of some underlying disorder, which is most commonly coronary heart disease. It is a tight, vice-like pain starting in the centre of the chest, often radiating to one or both arms and up the neck, and occurs in response to physical exertion or emotional stress which causes the heart to beat faster. The pain is transient and stops within seconds or minutes of stopping the exertion or resolving the emotional upset. Since angina is a symptom rather than a disease, the risks and treatments are those of the underlying condition; adopting self-help measures is a very important part of managing the condition. Angina is discussed in further detail in Chapter 8.

Heart attack

When one of the coronary arteries, that is already narrowed by atherosclerosis, becomes blocked by a blood clot, the blood supply to one portion of the heart muscle is cut off. The area deprived of blood then begins to die, unless the circulation is restored within a matter of hours, and is eventually replaced by scar tissue. If the size of the damaged area (called an infarct) is small, and if the heart's electrical conducting system, which determines the regularity of the heart beats, is not disturbed, your chances of survival are reasonably high.

A heart attack is also known as coronary thrombosis, cardiac infarction, or myocardial infarction (meaning, literally, destruction of the heart muscle). The symptoms are similar to angina, but occur at rest and last much longer. Heart attack is discussed in more detail in Chapter 9.

Rhythm disturbance

If coronary heart disease damages the heart's electrical pathways (see page 16) directly, or their function is disturbed by accumulation of certain chemicals

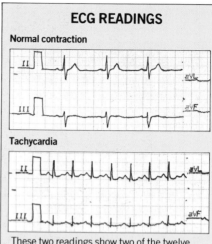

ECG READINGS

Normal contraction

Tachycardia

These two readings show two of the twelve traces taken when a doctor records heartbeat on an electrocardiogram, see page 37. The first ECG is one showing a normal heartbeat, the second reading indicates that the person has a fast heartbeat, tachycardia.

released during stress (see page 51) or by a heart attack, the electrical signals are upset and the regular rhythmic pace of the heart beat is disturbed. This is also known as heart irregularities, or arrythmia.

The pattern of heart irregularities can be recorded on an electrocardiogram (ECG), see page 37. They may just be odd ectopic beats (minor irregularities in an otherwise regular pulsation); more serious ventricular tachycardia (fast beating of the ventricles); or life-threatening ventricular fibrillation, in which the ventricles quiver like bags of worms instead of harmoniously contracting and acting as pumps. Heart irregularities and their treatment are described more fully in Chapter 9.

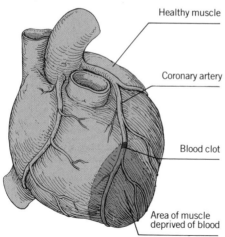

Coronary thrombosis

Healthy muscle

Coronary artery

Blood clot

Area of muscle deprived of blood

Cardiac arrest

As the name implies, the heart stops beating. When the heart stops, blood circulation to the brain ceases and the person becomes unconscious within a few seconds. It sometimes occurs out of the blue in a seemingly healthy person, who usually turns out to have un-diagnosed coronary heart disease. Occasionally, the serious heart irregu-larity known as ventricular fibrillation heralds the attack.

The prospects of recovery are good if resuscitation is started immediately, that is, mouth-to-mouth ventilation (the kiss of life) and external chest com-pression (see pages 101 to 104), and if it is kept going until help arrives and the patient is transferred to a hospital where more sophisticated resuscitation proce-dures and equipment are available.

WHEN TO CONSULT YOUR DOCTOR

Some of the conditions speak for them-selves; their severity is so obvious that, without doubt, you will contact your doctor. Others are more insidious and, unless they are checked, they will progress relentlessly. A condition such as high blood pressure can affect one in five adults, but it is a silent disease and does not produce symptoms unless it is well advanced or one of the possible complications has occurred.

In countries like the United States, people have regular – usually annual – medical check-ups. The National Health Service in the United Kingdom does not provide such check-ups. Surveys in both countries have shown that approximately half the people who have high blood pressure do not know they have it, either because their blood pressure has not been measured or their doctor has not informed them. Of the half that do know, only half are treated; and of the half that are treated, only half again are properly controlled. Clearly the situation is very unsatisfactory.

Make sure that you have your blood pressure measured. Most general prac-titioners have nurses in their practice so, if you do not want to waste your doctor's time because you are not actually ill, you can ask the nurse to take your blood pressure. Alternatively, if you have a medical department at work, have it measured there.

You should always consult your general practitioner if you have one or more of the following symptoms. There may be nothing wrong with your heart but it is better to let your doctor decide.

● **Breathlessness** Of all the possible symptoms of heart disease, breathless-ness is perhaps the most important. Breathlessness after exertion that formerly had no such effect is often the first indication of heart disease. It is noted for the first time after activities such as a brisk walk, after climbing stairs or while running to catch a bus.

● **Chest pain** Pain resulting from the heart is, of course, also important. This type of pain occurs in the centre of the chest and is a feeling of constriction or tightness. Not all pains in the chest are due to heart disease or angina, but you cannot be sure and it is always advisable to see a doctor.

● **Calf muscle pain** A cramp-like pain in one or both of your calves, which is felt only while walking, may be a symptom of peripheral vessel disease.

● **Fatigue** Weakness of the heart muscle, or a disease affecting one of the heart valves, may cause undue fatigue at the end of the day, or after an activity which formerly caused no such fatigue. Fatigue is also, however, a common symptom of many other conditions. If you are in any doubt, you should consult your doctor.

● **Swelling (oedema)** Swelling of the feet at the end of the day may be a manifestation of heart failure. In the early stages, this swelling usually disappears in the morning and reappears again in the evening. However, there are many other conditions which can produce such swelling.

● **Palpitations** Most patients feel that these must be a sure sign of heart disease. Actually they are not necessarily indicative of a serious disorder; it is just that you are conscious of the fact that your heart is beating rapidly. If you have recurrent attacks, however, you should see your doctor.

● **Missing heart beats** The feeling that your heart has missed a beat can be very frightening but does not necessarily signify heart disease. It may simply be due to an excess of coffee, tobacco or alcohol, and can often be remedied simply by cutting down on – or giving up – whatever was causing it. Only a doctor, however, can distinguish between the innocent variety and the type that is due to heart disease.

● **Headaches** If you do not usually suffer from headaches, they may be a sign of very high blood pressure. This can be detected only by having your blood pressure measured.

● **Sweating** When someone is in a state of medical shock, he perspires profusely. Sweating may also occur at the onset of a heart attack. However, sweating is often present in cases of cardiac neurosis.

● **Sore throat and throat infection** A sore throat, followed by a throat infection two or three weeks later, is a possible symptom of rheumatic fever, which may cause rheumatic heart disease. Rheumatic fever chiefly affects children between five and 15.

● **Inexplicable lump** An inexplicable lump, or a feeling of pressure anywhere in the body, but particularly in the abdomen, may indicate an aneurysm.

● **Increased passing of urine** A possible symptom of kidney failure, which can be caused by long-standing high blood pressure. Damaged kidneys can, in turn, raise blood pressure further. It is also a sign of diabetes.

● **Intensely itchy skin** Though there are many other causes of intensely itchy skin, this can be the result of kidney failure due to high blood pressure, particularly if accompanied by other symptoms such as loss of appetite, vomiting or increased passing of urine.

● **Feeling cold** Having cold hands and feet in spite of adequate heat, particularly if accompanied by chilblains, may be an indication of some circulatory disorder such as atherosclerosis. Constriction of the blood vessels means that blood is not able to carry enough warmth and energy to the extremities.

FALSE ALARMS

Some conditions are thought to be symptoms of heart disease, but they are more likely to be caused by something else. Nevertheless, if you are at all concerned, you should always consult your doctor.

● **Nose bleeds** These are commonly thought of as a sign of heart disease or of high blood pressure. However, although occasionally they can be, usually they are not.

● **Dizziness** Although this is a possible symptom of high blood pressure, in fact it is much more likely to be due to nervousness, or to a disorder of the nervous system, than to heart disease.

● **Fainting** Certain heart conditions such as a type of rhythm disturbance, can cause fainting attacks, but on the whole these are very rare. However, if you are having fainting attacks, your doctor will examine your heart.

3
Visiting the doctor

If you are worried about the health of your heart, or have experienced any of the symptoms mentioned on pages 29 to 30, do go to your doctor. Likewise, if you have a family history of heart disease, stroke or high blood pressure, talk to your doctor about it. There may well be nothing wrong with your heart, so the sooner your mind is put at rest the better.

History
First of all the doctor will ask you a lot of questions. Giving him an accurate medical history is always of the utmost importance – sometimes more important even than a thorough medical examination. For example, a doctor is more likely to distinguish whether or not a chest pain is angina (see page 27) entirely from your medical and personal history. He will want to know your age, what your symptoms are, how long you have had them, what brings them on, what makes them worse and what relieves them. It is also useful for him to know if there is any family history of high blood pressure, heart attacks, strokes or diabetes.

If you have any personal or emotional problems, do discuss them freely with your doctor – they may have a bearing on your symptoms. You can confide in him even your most intimate problems, and you can rest assured that your confidence will not be breached.

Examination
The doctor will then check your weight, listen to your heart and lungs with a stethoscope, take your pulse and blood pressure, and examine the rest of your body. He may also look into your eyes with an instrument called an ophthalmoscope. The reason for this is that the blood vessels on the retina are the only ones in the body that can easily be seen and they give the doctor a useful indication of the state of the blood vessels.

Examining the retina
Your doctor will shine a light into your eye with an instrument called an ophthalmoscope. The photographs below show how clearly she can see the blood vessels.

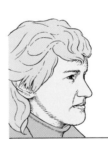

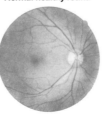

Normal healthy retina

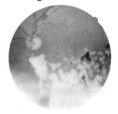

Retina with severely damaged blood vessels

MEASURING BLOOD PRESSURE

The single most important test in the campaign against heart disease is measuring blood pressure: it is quick, cheap and painless, with no side-effects. Blood pressure is measured with a simple device called a sphygmomanometer (from the Greek *Sphygmos*, meaning pulse) and sometimes referred to as a blood pressure cuff. It works by applying pressure to the main artery in the arm (the brachial artery) and gradually releasing it. A stethoscope is usually required to listen to the sounds produced by oscillation, or vibration, of the artery walls as the pressure in the cuff is reduced and the blood flows through the artery again.

How is blood pressure measured?

First of all, you will be asked to roll your sleeve right up to your shoulder. Your doctor will wrap the cuff around your arm just above the elbow and feel for your wrist pulse (the radial pulse) with his fingers. He will then inflate the cuff until the mercury column reads 20 to 25mmHg above the point where the pulse can no longer be felt. This

---

EQUIPMENT FOR MEASURING BLOOD PRESSURE

Every sphygmomanometer consists of a scale on which the pressure units are written in millimetres of mercury (mmHg), a cuff containing an inflatable rubber bag with two tubes – one which leads to the measuring scale and the other to an inflation bulb. There is a valve situated between the bulb and the tubing. the adjustment of which controls the deflation of the rubber bag.

There are several types of sphygmomanometer in general use today, the most commonly used being the mercury and aneroid kinds. The first one has a vertical mercury column and works on the simple principle of balancing liquids with pressure; the other, "aneroid" type – so called from the Greek meaning literally "not fluid" – has a compact, circular dial.

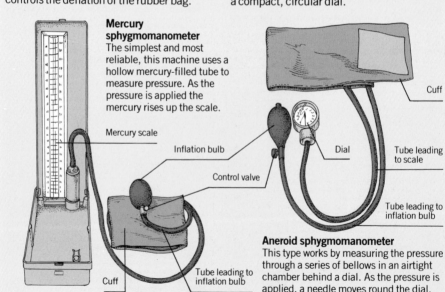

Mercury sphygmomanometer
The simplest and most reliable, this machine uses a hollow mercury-filled tube to measure pressure. As the pressure is applied the mercury rises up the scale.

Mercury scale

Inflation bulb

Control valve

Cuff

Tube leading to inflation bulb

Cuff

Dial

Tube leading to scale

Tube leading to inflation bulb

Aneroid sphygmomanometer
This type works by measuring the pressure through a series of bellows in an airtight chamber behind a dial. As the pressure is applied, a needle moves round the dial.

simultaneously compresses the brachial artery in the arm (see page 19), and shuts off the blood flow through it.

Your doctor will then place the stethoscope over the main artery in the front of the elbow and just below the cuff, and gradually release the air from the cuff, while watching the mercury column slowly falling. When the air pressure in the cuff falls just below the maximum amount of pressure in the brachial artery, your doctor will hear a sudden thudding sound through the stethoscope, which is the sound of the artery wall oscillating as the blood is forced through it by the heart. He will then make a note of this level, which is the systolic pressure (see page 18). Your doctor will then continue to release air from the cuff until the pressure in the cuff equals the pressure inside the artery. When this happens the artery stops oscillating and the blood flows steadily through the artery. The doctor will make a note of the reading on the scale at this point – the diastolic pressure (see page 18).

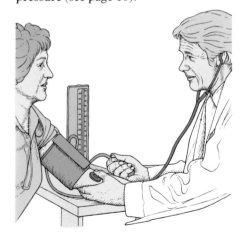

Having your blood pressure measured
This is a very simple procedure that can be carried out by your doctor or the nurse. It is very important because it gives an insight into the state of your heart and blood vessels.

What the reading means

Blood pressure is always expressed in millimetres of mercury, written as mmHg, irrespective of the type of sphygmomanometer used. It should be emphasized here that there is no clearly defined blood pressure level above which pressure is too high or below which it is too low; the figures vary from one person to another. Having said that, however, the normal blood pressure under relaxed conditions will probably be between 100 and 140mmHg systolic and between 60 and 90 diastolic; written as 100/60mmHg or 140/90mmHg. It is more likely to be in the upper end of this range as you get older.

Your blood pressure will not be taken immediately if you have just:
● Done anything strenuous, such as climbing the stairs
● Drunk a cup of coffee
● Eaten a heavy meal
● Smoked a cigarette
● Been emotionally upset.
These factors all cause a temporary rise in the reading, which will therefore be higher than your normal blood pressure when you are at rest.

It is not unusual for blood pressure to rise temporarily as high as 250mmHg/130mmHg after strenuous exercise or during emotional upset. Because of this, even if your doctor does obtain a high blood pressure reading on the first examination, he will be loathe to jump to conclusions. A misleadingly high reading can be obtained if you are in a hurry, nervous, anxious, or if you have recently exerted yourself, so he will probably want you to rest for half an hour or make another appointment, so that he can test your blood pressure again. High blood pressure, and what it can involve, is discussed in greater detail in the high blood pressure chapter (see pages 66 to 79).

THE DISCOVERY OF BLOOD PRESSURE

An English clergyman from Kent, the Reverend Stephen Hales, was the first person, in 1732, to realize what blood pressure was. He fitted a vertical brass tube into a cut in the main artery of a horse's left leg and noticed that the blood level in the tube rose to more than 2m (8ft) above the level of its heart.

It took almost one hundred years before a French medical student, Poiseuille, thought of connecting a mercury-filled U-tube to an artery. Because mercury is 13.6 times heavier than water, the column in the tube rose to a much lesser height and it became possible to measure blood pressure indoors. Since this time, the height of displacement of the mercury column, measured in millimetres of mercury (mmHg), has been the standard way of measuring blood pressure.

It was not until 1896, however, that an Italian physiologist called Riva-Rocci first developed a sphygmomanometer, versions of which are still used today. For the first time it became possible to measure blood pressure accurately and easily without cutting an artery.

The sphygmomanometer on its own, however, was capable of measuring only the systolic pressure (see page 18). Then, finally, in 1905, a Russian physician, Nicolai Korotkoff, discovered that a stethoscope, placed over the main artery of the arm, allowed him to listen to the sounds of pulsation through the artery that indicate both systolic and diastolic pressure (see page 18).

FURTHER TESTS

If the doctor feels from your history and a simple examination that your heart, circulation and blood pressure are all normal, he may do nothing else. If he cannot explain your symptoms, he may carry out a few more simple tests.

The tests described here are those most commonly used if the doctor does not suspect anything serious. If the results indicate any potentially serious problem, he will refer you to a specialist who will probably conduct further tests.

You must remember that only your doctor can tell you at this stage which are the best tests for you. The point of discussing the various tests here is to make you aware of what types are available. They may not all be indicated or desirable in your case.

URINE TESTS

If your doctor suspects kidney disease or diabetes, both of which are often linked with heart disease, he will carry out a urine test. Examination of urine for abnormalities is one of the oldest diagnostic tests.

A lot of urine tests are carried out in the doctor's surgery by dipping small strips of paper impregnated with various chemicals into a specimen of urine. The chemicals react with the urine, and any change in the colour produced is then compared with the standardized colour chart given on the bottle containing the strips. The test detects not only the presence of any abnormal constituents in the urine, but also the approximate quantity of any abnormal substance.

The kidneys act as a filtering system, removing waste chemicals, such as urea, and excess water from the blood travelling through them and passing them out of the body in urine. They also reabsorb other substances, initially filtered out. The presence or absence of certain substances in your urine gives an indication of the state of your kidneys and circulatory system.

The presence of sugar in the urine may indicate diabetes (see page 47), although sometimes certain other substances, such as vitamin C, may produce a falsely positive test. The presence of protein, if temporary, may indicate an infection, but if its presence continues, it may indicate that the kidney is damaged to such an extent that it is leaking protein. The presence of blood and other abnormal substances may also be detected by this type of simple strip dipping.

In addition, a urine sample may be sent to a laboratory for more elaborate tests. For this purpose, you will be asked to provide a sample of mid-stream urine (MSU) in a sterilized container. It is looked at under a microscope for the presence of any abnormalities, and may also be cultured, in order to see if there are bacteria present. If there are any significant abnormalities, you may be referred to hospital for further tests of kidney function, such as a special kidney X-ray.

BLOOD TESTS

If heart disease is suspected, a blood sample is taken from a vein in front of the elbow and sent for various tests.

Anaemia

One of these tests is for anaemia, a condition in which the level of haemoglobin, the red pigment in the blood, is too low. Haemoglobin is the most important component of the red blood cells, which combines with oxygen in the lungs and carries it through the body (see page 12). The level of haemoglobin, the total number of red and white cells, the size and

shape of red cells and the proportion of different types of white cells all provide information on your state of health.

Anaemia can restrict the supply of blood to the heart and so aggravate angina (see page 27), as well as the symptoms of heart failure (see page 24). It always requires further investigation and correction, which is usually through medication or diet. For example, there may be a fault in the production of haemoglobin itself, or the production of the red blood cells. The production of haemoglobin is dependent on a daily intake of iron. Lack of vitamin B_{12} in the diet can result in defective red blood cells.

Kidney function

Another blood test is sometimes carried out to assess the function of the kidneys, and the levels of various salts (electrolytes) and waste products, mainly urea and creatinine, in the blood. If the kidneys are functioning properly, levels of these waste products are kept low; but if the kidneys are not functioning properly, waste products are not excreted in the urine as efficiently as they should be and therefore accumulate in the blood.

Salt level

Levels of various salts in the blood such as sodium and potassium are also measured. If kidney function is disturbed, the level of potassium may be raised. On the other hand, a very low level of potassium may indicate depletion due to diuretics (drugs which increase the flow of urine), which are prescribed for high blood pressure (see page 73) and congestive heart failure, or it may indicate some hormonal imbalance in the body. The importance of maintaining correct sodium and potassium levels is discussed in greater detail in Chapter 10.

Blood fat levels

If you are suspected of having atherosclerosis or coronary artery disease, or some member of your family has recently died of a heart attack and was under the age of 55 years, the blood fat levels of the plasma (the liquid part of the blood from which blood cells have been removed) will be measured. You will be asked to fast for at least ten hours before the test. This ensures the most accurate reading and prevents it from being affected by anything you have eaten or drunk. Small amounts of blood fat – cholesterol and triglycerides – are essential for certain bodily functions, but high levels are believed to be implicated in atherosclerosis (see Chapter 6) and thus in coronary artery disease (see pages 27 and 63). Blood fats are measured in units called millimols per litre. Although there is no definitive amount of cholesterol that should be present, levels above 7.2mmol per litre of cholesterol and 1.2mmol per litre of triglycerides are considered abnormal.

Blood sugar levels

Diabetics often have a raised blood sugar level (see page 47), so your fasting level of blood sugar is particularly likely to be measured if you have a family history of diabetes. A high level of sugar can increase the chances of having heart and blood vessel disease.

CHEST X-RAY

If you have been diagnosed as having high blood pressure, coronary heart disease or heart failure, you may also be asked to have a chest X-ray, which is a completely painless procedure, just like having a photograph taken. It provides the doctor with vital information about the size of your heart. The heart is a muscular organ and, if it has been pumping blood at a higher pressure

than normal for a prolonged period, the muscle develops, or enlarges, to cope with the extra work. This enlarging of the heart is not only a sign of an overworked heart but it also puts extra strain on the coronary arteries because the larger muscle needs more oxygen and nutrients. Even if an abnormal increase in the size of the heart is not expected, your doctor will still arrange for you to

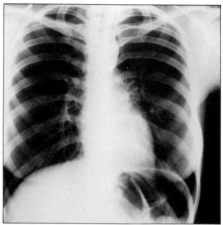

Above **Normal heart** *Below* **Enlarged heart**

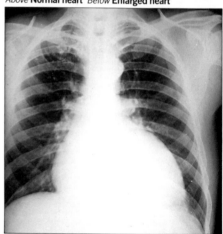

Chest X-rays
The heart shows up as the area of solid white near the bottom of the rib cage. Here you can see quite clearly the difference between a normal and enlarged heart.

have an X-ray so that it can be compared with future ones.

In addition to the size of the heart, a chest X-ray can show up any congestion in the lungs, which may be a sign that the heart is not pumping as well as it should (congestive heart failure see page 24). The arteries are not visible on X-ray, whether they are healthy or not, so the diagnosis of atherosclerosis relies largely on a process of deduction.

ELECTROCARDIOGRAM

An electrocardiogram (ECG) is the tracing of the electrical activity of the heart and is usually performed in hospital, though some general practices and specialists have their own electrocardiograph. It is a completely painless procedure in which electrodes, in the form of plastic or metal discs, are placed on the ankles, wrists and various parts of the chest wall and are connected by wires to the recording machine. Twelve different tracings, which view the heart's electrical activity from different angles, are usually taken. As the heart beats and relaxes, the signals of the heart's electrical activities are picked up and the pattern is recorded.

An ECG taken while you are at rest can tell a good deal about the state of your heart. It may indicate if high blood pressure has produced any strain on the heart. It can also tell if your heart is beating regularly or irregularly, fast or slow. Certain patterns may reveal a poor blood supply through the coronary arteries, which is indicative of coronary heart disease. Conversely, a normal ECG does not necessarily mean that the coronary arteries are perfectly normal. A previously unnoticed heart attack may be picked up by an ECG, and in fact the most important use of the ECG is to reveal whether an acute chest pain, lasting more than a few minutes, was due to a heart attack. You may need several ECGs to get a diagnosis.

Vecterocardiogram

A variation on the ECG is the vecterocardiogram (VCG). It is performed in exactly the same way as the ECG, except that the electrical activity is shown in the form of loops (vectors), which can be watched on a screen, printed on paper or photographed. It provides a three-dimensional view of a single heart beat.

ECG tracings

On a normal ECG, the tracings show a small smooth curve at the beginning of the heartbeat, this is the spread of electric current through the atrial muscle, followed by a sharp peak as the electric current passes into the ventricles. Another smooth upward curve follows as the ventricles relax. The amount of activity should be same with each heartbeat. The first series of tracings show normal, regular heartbeat; the second set show a much faster and more uneven heartbeat, a condition known as tachycardia.

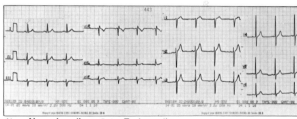

Above **Normal readings** *Below* **Tachycardia**

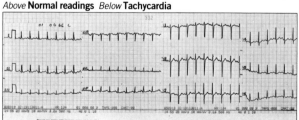

4
Risk factors

During the last 30 to 40 years, a number of personal, social and behavioural characteristics have been identified as increasing the risks of atherosclerosis and coronary heart disease. These characteristics are known as risk factors.

Age, gender, high blood pressure, a high level of blood cholesterol and cigarette smoking have all been shown to have a strong link with coronary heart disease and are the major risk factors. Many doctors now also believe that there are certain categories of personality, prone to aggressive competitive and hostile behaviour patterns, which constitute a major coronary risk factor. These are dealt with in Chapter 5, Stress: a neglected risk factor.

Modifiable and unmodifiable risks

Diet, obesity, lack of exercise and diabetes are all considered to be minor but important risk factors. And then there is the role played by stress, resulting from various psychological, social, occupational and cultural factors; these factors are considered minor because of the problems of definition and measurement. For details, see Chapter 5.

Some of the risk factors, such as age and gender, merely describe who we are and are considered as unmodifiable risk factors, because we cannot do anything about them. Other risk factors are considered "potentially modifiable". It is important to remember, however, that all of these risk factors merely indicate an increased chance of developing the disease. They do not necessarily *cause* coronary heart disease, and it is impossible to predict who will succumb to the disease.

Presence of risk factors

By and large, the presence of one major risk factor doubles the average chance of having a heart attack; two major risk factors quadruple the chances; and three major risk factors increase the risk by nine times. Minor risk factors do not increase the risk as much, but again, the greater the number of factors the greater the risk. There is also a considerable overlap between modifiable and non-modifiable risk factors. Most people do not have all the risk factors discussed here, but the chances are that you will have at least one of them.

Most of the preventive efforts advised by doctors so far have been aimed at reducing blood pressure, blood cholesterol level, cigarette smoking and obesity, while encouraging increased physical activity. Unfortunately, these risk factors account for only half of the heart attacks, so that reducing them does not mean that coronary heart disease will be eliminated. It is for this reason that other potential risk factors are examined here. Turn to the self-help section, pages 124 to 186 for advice on minimizing your risks.

UNMODIFIABLE RISK FACTORS

These are the risk factors that are part of our genetic make-up, either because they are inherited, for example, a family history of heart problems, or because of age or gender, which cannot be altered.

The ageing process

As we get older, the efficiency of our cardiovascular system declines, and the chances of something going wrong with it are increased.

Approximately 40 per cent of deaths in men between the ages of 45 and 64 years in the developed world are due to coronary heart disease. The death rate from this disease in men, between the ages of 35 and 44 years, doubled in England and Wales between 1952-1972, and there have even been cases, albeit rare, of people having a heart attack in their twenties. The fact that coronary heart disease is not an inevitable consequence of ageing is shown by the disparity in the number of deaths in similar age groups, see below.

Gender

Coronary heart disease is often called a "disease of men" because, compared with women of the same age, men are three to five times more likely to die of it under the age of 50 but no one really knows why. Over the age of 50 or after the menopause, however, more and more women tend to have heart attacks and the gap between the sexes closes. Strokes tend to occur in both sexes in equal numbers at any age.

Inherited factors

There is no doubt that heart and circulatory disease runs in families. If your parents, grandparents, brothers or sisters have had a heart attack or stroke, your chances of having one are higher than if you come from a family without any such problems. What is not certain is how these tendencies are inherited. Is it the presence of a particular gene that increases the risk, or is it the absence of a particular gene which might normally play a protective role?

There is no doubt that some of the risk factors – such as high blood pressure and an extremely high level of blood cholesterol – are partly inherited, while an increased tendency to smoke, over-eat and drink while taking less

DEATH RATES PER MILLION IN ENGLAND AND WALES, 1979							
Cause of death	Age group:	25–34	35–44	45–54	55–64	65–74	All ages
All causes	Male	971	1993	6645	18788	48513	12437
	Female	559	1358	4138	9910	25268	11703
Neoplasms	Male	167	440	1774	5676	13179	2890
	Female	183	620	2010	4110	6934	2396
Cardiovascular diseases	Male	135	760	3512	9785	25087	6128
	Female	70	276	1122	3750	12918	6014
Coronary heart disease	Male	65	551	2762	7288	16266	3781
	Female	15	90	531	2023	6790	2581
Accidents/ violence/poison	Male	485	454	461	582	710	506
	Female	153	194	299	348	557	359

DEATHS FROM CORONARY HEART DISEASE

The graph below, prepared from figures published by the World Health Organisation, shows clearly the change in the number of deaths from coronary heart disease in different countries. In the United States and Finland, where health consciousness is most prevalent, the number of deaths has fallen dramatically. The figures for England and Wales are disappointing. In Japan, where the rates have always been low, they continue to decline in spite of a recent increase in dietary fat.

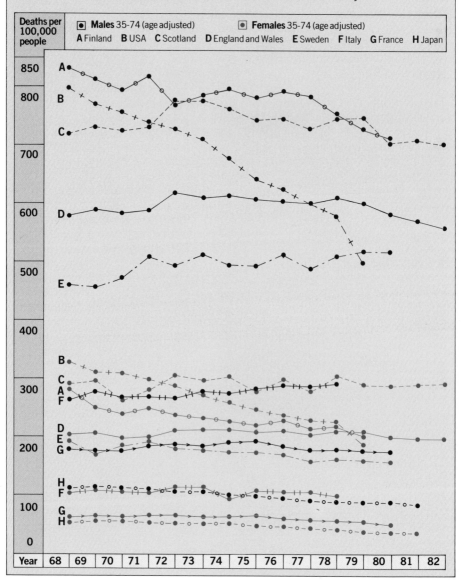

exercise might be the result of shared environments and are modifiable.

If there is a family history of heart disease, stroke or high blood pressure, you should talk to your doctor about this and ask him how often you and members of your family – including teenagers – should have your blood pressure checked. He will probably suggest you have it measured every two years, or more frequently if it shows any sign of rising. Not all children in a family where there is a history of high blood pressure will develop it, however. In addition, people without a family history of hypertension may be affected.

Family environment

This is considered an unmodifiable risk factor because families not only share their genes, they also share a common environment – although this could in theory be considered modifiable. Family members living together, eat together and interact with each other, and the effects of similar social, cultural environments from an early age are important ones. In favour of this environmental theory is the observation that high blood pressure often occurs in both husband and wife, while only one of identical twins develops the disease if separated soon after birth and brought up in a different environment.

A stressful home life – squabbles and destructive criticism between spouses, unreasonable demands from parents, and unhealthy rivalries between siblings – can all increase the chances of heart attacks and high blood pressure.

Racial differences

High blood pressure is more prevalent in blacks, particularly women living in westernized countries. It occurs at an earlier age than in whites, is often more severe and has a greater chance of developing complications.

The death rate from diseases related to high blood pressure in certain parts of the United States is 10 to 20 times higher in blacks compared with the rest of the population. High blood pressure is more prevalent among those living in high-stress areas than in those living in a low-stress area. (Stress is rated on the basis of crime rate, family income, level of education, level of unemployment, divorce and separation rates, density of population and population mobility.)

POTENTIALLY MODIFIABLE FACTORS

These are the factors which increase the chance of heart disease developing but which we can control, thereby reducing the possibility of heart disease.

CIGARETTE SMOKING

This increases the chances of having not only coronary heart disease (see page 27) but also peripheral vessel disease (see page 26) and lung disorders such as chronic bronchitis, emphysema, asthma and lung cancer. Coronary heart disease is the most significant of these diseases as a relatively larger number of people are affected by it than, say, lung cancer. More than half of deaths in smokers are due to cardiovascular disease.

Although the overall risk in smokers is about double that of non-smokers of the same age, gender and other risk factor status, the adverse effect of smoking is far greater in young men and women under the age of 30, increasing their risk up to 10 times, while its effect in older people (who have a higher risk anyway) is less dramatic. Among British doctors who smoke, the death rate is five times higher in the 35-44 year age group, and four times higher in the 45-54 year age group compared with doctors who do not smoke.

The effect of smoking is also dose-related which means that the more you smoke, the greater the likelihood of dying from coronary heart disease. Those who start smoking before the age of 20 and those who smoke 20 or more cigarettes a day have eight times the risk compared with non-smokers, and twice the risk compared with those who smoke fewer than ten cigarettes a day. Heavy smokers are also five times more likely to die a sudden death. Smokers of pipes and cigars are, on the whole, at less risk because they do not usually inhale, but they are still at greater risk than non-smokers.

How smoking affects the heart

The adverse effects of smoking on the heart are due to carbon monoxide and nicotine. Carbon monoxide inhaled in cigarette smoke combines with haemoglobin in the red blood cells to form carboxyhaemoglobin reducing the amount of oxygen available to the heart muscle (see page 143). Nicotine stimulates the production of the stress hormone adrenaline and its close relative noradrenaline, both of which increase

the heart rate and cause a temporary rise in blood pressure. Both carbon monoxide and nicotine also increase the stickiness of platelets and thus the likelihood of clot formation, and damage the lining of the blood vessels leaving them more prone to atherosclerosis. However, the precise reason for this is not yet clearly understood.

There are a few anomalies: smoking has increased among women in Switzerland, Sweden and the United Kingdom, yet deaths among women from coronary heart disease have decreased in all of these countries. In addition, smoking is very common in Japan, yet the incidence of coronary heart disease there is the lowest known in the world. The harmful effects of smoking are, however, undeniable and the observed discrepancies are therefore likely to be attributed to the presence or absence of other risk factors and possible protective factors.

Smoking causes a temporary rise in blood pressure rather than chronic, or permanent, high blood pressure. If, on the other hand, you have high blood pressure or a raised level of cholesterol in your blood, smoking is likely to compound the risk of coronary heart disease. Thus if a person with high blood pressure has twice the risk of coronary heart disease, the risk is quadrupled if that person also smokes.

CORONARY HEART DISEASE AND SMOKING

Over 1 pack a day		
½ to 1 pack a day		
Non-smoker		
Low	1½ times	2 times

Risk of heart disease (source, see page 192)

HIGH BLOOD PRESSURE

Until a few years ago, it was the general belief than an increase in blood pressure with advancing age was normal. This was based on population studies in which it was noticed that average blood pressures were found to be higher in older age groups. It is now known that blood pressure does not *have* to rise with age. Indeed, studies both in the United States and in Britain indicate that, in a substantial proportion of people, blood pressure does not rise with age. Those who start out with a higher than average blood pressure, however, have been found to have five times the risk of developing high blood pressure compared with those whose initial blood pressure was in the lower range of normal.

Under the age of 45, more men have high blood pressure than women; after the age of 45, there is a steep rise in the number of women with high blood pressure; after the age of 55, women overtake men. The causes for this disparity are not really clear, but it is possible that women are protected by female hormones during their reproductive life. Different factors are likely to be operative in men. For example, they are more likely to be under considerable stress at work while their families' needs are greatest. Women who suffer from coronary heart disease are, in the main, more likely to be smokers, breadwinners and to take the contraceptive pill.

How does it affect the circulation?

High blood pressure is one of the major risk factors for atherosclerosis and coronary heart disease. Population studies consistently show that raised blood pressure is a powerful predictor of coronary heart disease for that population, though not for each individual.

Although people with severe hypertension are far more likely to have a stroke or heart failure, the number of people with such severe hypertension is relatively few. Even a mild rise in blood pressure on the other hand, is associated with a slightly increased risk of coronary heart disease. Since 70 per cent of all people with high blood pressure fall into the mild category (between 90-105mmHg diastolic and 140-160mmHg

systolic), mild high blood pressure is the greatest contributor to the total number of people who get coronary heart disease.

A study involving 18,000 male civil servants in London in the seventies showed that two-thirds of all coronary deaths occurred in people with a diastolic blood pressure of less than 105mmHg. Similar results have been found in Wales, Scotland and the United States. Recently, however, considerable publicity has brought this to the attention of both the public and physicians in the United States and, as a result, more and more people are having their blood pressure measured and controlled. The state of affairs in the United Kingdom is less satisfactory, since unfortunately, a lot of people with mild hypertension are unaware that they have it.

The link with other risk factors

The effect of high blood pressure as a risk factor in the development of coronary heart disease is compounded by cigarette smoking and by a raised level of blood cholesterol. Thus, if the risk is double for a smoker compared with a non-smoker, it is quadrupled for a smoker who also has high blood pressure, and the risk continues to rise as the level of blood pressure increases.

High blood pressure is discussed in more detail in Chapter 7.

BLOOD FATS

The most significant fats – or, in medical terms, lipids – in the blood are cholesterol and triglycerides. There is no precise level beyond which they are considered abnormal but, on the whole, the higher level the greater the risk. The level is influenced by fat in the diet, particularly that of animal origin, as well as by too low an intake of fibre, by too much sugar, alcohol and coffee, and by obesity, the contraceptive pill, physical inactivity and emotional stress.

The body also produces its own fat (including cholesterol) independently of diet (see page 128), and the level of fats in the blood is also affected by the way our kidneys get rid of excess fats. What we eat, however, is the most important and easily modifiable factor. A certain amount of fat, in the form of essential fatty acids, is necessary in order to maintain the body, to enable production of certain hormones and enzymes as well as for warmth and energy, but if it is eaten in excess, it is deposited in the arteries as part of the process of atherosclerosis and thus narrows down the blood vessels.

Cholesterol

The level of fat that is most commonly measured in the blood is the cholesterol level. While a certain amount is essential for metabolic and other energy-controlling procedures, population studies comparing communities in different parts of the world have shown that a rise in the average level of cholesterol is associated with a higher rate of coronary heart disease.

Communities with a low level of cholesterol in the blood, ranging from 3.9 to 5.2 millimols per litre (150-180 milligrams per decilitre), have a much lower risk. This is the case in Japan, in some Greek islands, in rural Italy and in other Mediterranean countries.

The levels in some industrialized countries, on the other hand, are higher, ranging upwards from 6.4 millimols per litre (250 milligrams per decilitre), and carry a considerably higher risk of developing coronary heart disease. These countries include the United States, Britain and Finland In the middle ranges of cholesterol

CORONARY HEART DISEASE AND CHOLESTEROL LEVEL

Blood cholesterol level

Blood cholesterol level	Low	1½ times	2 times	2½
Over 6.4 mmol/litre				
5.63 – 6.4				
5.01 – 5.63				
Under 5.01				

Risk of heart disease (source, see page 192)

levels the relationship between the level and the risk is not so clear cut and depends on many other factors.

Some long-term community studies, both in the United Kingdom and the United States, have shown that the individual's level of blood cholesterol is a major predictor of further coronary heart disease. In a long-running population study in the town of Framingham, Massachusetts, for example, some 5,000 healthy adults were examined for several risk factors, including their blood cholesterol level, and followed up for 20 years; those who subsequently developed coronary heart disease had a substantially higher cholesterol level at the initial examination. Other studies confirm these findings.

Recent research has shown that some cholesterol in the blood is necessary. It circulates in the bloodstream combined with chemical carriers known as lipoproteins, which vary in density and size. Low density lipoproteins (LDL) and very low density lipoproteins (VLDL), carry cholesterol into the tissues, so accelerating the rate of atherosclerosis. High density lipoproteins (HDL), on the other hand, seem to remove it again; they have more protein, less cholesterol, and are thought to be protective. This is explained in more detail in Chapter 6, Atherosclerosis. When blood fat levels are tested, it is normally the total cholesterol level which is taken. There is evidence, however, to suggest that measuring the ratio of LDL to HDL may be a better indication of a person's risk of future heart disease. This may also explain why some people with an apparently normal cholesterol level, develop coronary heart disease.

It is important to recognize that the number of individuals with a very high level of cholesterol (7.2mmol per litre or above) is low and, although their relative risk is high, the majority of deaths occur in people with only mild to moderate levels of blood cholesterol (5.6-7.2mmol per litre). This is so because, quite simply, there are many more people in this category. Extremely high levels of blood cholesterol (above 11mmol per litre) tend to run in families; the condition is known as *familiar hypercholesterolaemia*. Members of such families are prone to premature coronary heart disease.

So how can you find out if your own cholesterol level is raised? A simple blood test is the answer (see page 36). If you have a family history of early heart disease, do ask your doctor if he thinks

you and your family should have your cholesterol levels checked.

The risk associated with a raised level of blood cholesterol is compounded by high blood pressure and cigarette smoking. The diagram below clearly illustrates the effect of various combinations of risk factors when a single cut-off point is used to separate "high" blood cholesterol levels from those that are "not high". High blood pressure is also arbitrarily separated from normal blood pressure. When risk factors are combined, the total risk is greater than the sum of each one taken singly.

Triglycerides

A high level of triglycerides is an additional risk factor in communities with a moderate to high incidence of coronary heart disease. Its effect is not as great as that of cholesterol in the blood and may, in part, be due to an associated increase in cholesterol.

Raised levels are not usually found in anyone under 30. The levels are increased by obesity, diabetes, and an excessive intake of alcohol and sugar. It is usual nowadays for a doctor to check triglycerides whenever a blood test is carried out to check the cholesterol. Levels of 1.2 millimols per litre or more are considered to be high.

CORONARY HEART DISEASE AND MULTIPLE FACTORS

High blood pressure, high cholesterol and cigarettes

High cholesterol and cigarettes

Cigarettes

None of these

| Low | 1½ times | 3 times | 5 times |

Risk of heart disease (source, see page 192)

45

DIET

There are certain dietary risk factors which it is well within your power to do something about. A healthy eating plan is outlined in Chapter 10.

Saturated fat

Communities in which people eat food containing large amounts of cholesterol and saturated fats have a higher risk of atherosclerosis, high blood pressure and coronary heart disease than those communities in which less of these foods is eaten. Both cholesterol and saturated fat tend to increase the level of cholesterol in the blood (see page 128).

Foods high in cholesterol include eggs; offal (liver, kidney, brain, heart, sweetbread); and shellfish (prawns, shrimps). Saturated fats are hard and mostly of animal origin. Foods high in saturated fats include fatty red meats (beef, lamb and pork); certain meat products (sausages, hot dogs, salami, bacon, pâté); dairy products (hard or full-fat cheese, milk, cream, ice cream and butter); and cooking fats (lard, dripping, suet and margarine, except for soft margarine labelled as high in polyunsaturated fats).

Sugar

There is some evidence that a high consumption of sugar increases the risk of coronary heart disease or even heart attacks (see page 27) and peripheral vessel disease (see page 26), though no one knows quite why this should be so. The evidence, in any case, is confounded by the fact that those who eat a lot of sugar also tend to consume a large amount of butter and cream and are more likely to be smokers. Because of this it is difficult to separate the effect of sugar from that of fat consumption and cigarette smoking. In countries such as Venezuela and Mauritius and in the Caribbean, on the other hand, a large amount of sugar is consumed, but coronary heart disease is low.

Sugar tends to increase blood triglycerides, but there is no evidence that it also increases cholesterol. What is certain, however, is that it contains a lot of calories without having any other nutritional value and is therefore likely to contribute to obesity. Did you know, for example, that two teaspoonsful of sugar contain 50 calories, which is the same as in 100g (4oz) of fresh peas?

Salt

Table salt, the salt we are most familiar with, is sodium chloride, also known as sodium salt. Although not directly implicated in coronary heart disease, sodium salt may contribute to the development of high blood pressure. A very strict salt-free diet of rice and fruit was the only available treatment for high blood pressure before drug treatments became available in the 1950s.

Geographic variations in blood pressure are often explained in terms of salt intake. Eskimoes, for example, consume 4g ($\frac{1}{10}$oz) of salt per day and have the lowest average blood pressure.

Not everyone who consumes large amounts of salt, however, is going to develop high blood pressure. It would appear that some people are more sensitive to salt than others and this sensitivity is probably inherited.

Another salt, potassium salt is also needed by the body. A delicate balance of sodium and potassium salt is essential for kidney function (see pages 130 to 132). There is some evidence that increased consumption of potassium salt may actually reduce blood pressure.

Alcohol

In moderation – up to two drinks a day (see page 138) – alcohol does no harm and is even thought to be beneficial, though again no one knows why this should be so. More than three to four drinks a day, however, may well cause problems. It has been shown, for example, that both men and women who have three or more drinks per day have higher blood pressure. They are also more likely to be obese, to smoke, to drink a lot of coffee, and not to eat a nutritious, well-balanced diet. Alcohol also increases the chances of athero-sclerosis and raised levels of cholesterol and triglycerides.

Coffee

Although coffee has been incriminated in coronary heart disease, the evidence for this is conflicting. Excessive coffee drinking (5 to 6 cups or more per day) is likely to be associated with a raised level of blood cholesterol and the chance of having heart irregularity (rhythm disturbance). Coffee can cause a transient rise in blood pressure because of its high caffeine content.

Obesity

People who are obese have an excess of fat stored under the skin or in the chest and abdomen. Fat is the energy store of the body and is derived not only from the fat you eat but also from the carbo-hydrate and protein. If you eat more calories than you burn up, the excess will be stored as fat in the body. If you are overweight, your heart has to work harder to supply blood to all that extra fat, whereas if you lose weight, this will make more blood available and release enough fuel for the body's work.

If you can pinch more than 2.5cm (1in) of skinfold over the abdomen or under the upper arm, the chances are that you are overweight. Alternatively, if your weight is 20 per cent above the normal for your height and body frame (see the height/weight chart on page 133), you are considered to be over-weight. By this definition, however, one man in five and one woman in three in our society is, to some extent, obese.

There is no doubt in the minds of the public that to be obese is to increase the risk of having coronary heart disease. Yet population studies have shown that if blood pressure and the level of blood cholesterol are both normal and you do not smoke, then the risk associated with being overweight is negligible. The reason that so much emphasis has been put on obesity is that it is often associ-ated with other risk factors, such as high blood pressure, diabetes, a sedentary way of life, and a raised level of blood cholesterol and triglycerides.

A recent long-term study in Sweden showed that it is not obesity *per se* but the distribution of fat that is more important. The so-called pot-bellies, with a waist to hip measurement in the ratio of 1.0 or more in men and 0.8 in women, are four times more likely to suffer from a stroke or heart attack.

DIABETES

In order to utilize blood sugar as a fuel for energy, we require insulin, a hormone produced by the pancreas. With diabetes, there is a deficiency of insulin, either partial or total. As a result, the sugar level in the blood rises, which may damage the blood vessels.

There are two broad categories of diabetes. One is *juvenile diabetes*, a genetically inherited condition occur-ring in children and young adults in whom the pancreas almost completely fails to produce insulin. This disease is severe and treatment has to be given in the form of insulin injections. The other variety tends to occur in older and obese people and is called *maturity-onset diabetes*, in which inadequate insulin is produced. This form of the disease is less severe and is generally controlled either by a low carbohydrate diet or, in some cases, a combination of this and sugar-reducing drugs taken by mouth. Occasionally, insulin injections may be necessary, although this is rare. This type of diabetes tends to run in families.

The evidence regarding diabetes as an independent risk factor is conflicting, although studies have shown an association between diabetes and an increased susceptibility to atherosclerosis. It is believed that at least part of this association is due to other risk factors usually found in diabetic patients. Maturity-onset diabetic patients tend to have a higher level of blood cholesterol, obesity and high blood pressure.

In Western countries, diabetic men have a two to three times greater risk, and women a five to six times greater risk, of developing coronary heart disease. Half of all diabetics, in fact, die of coronary heart disease. Diabetics are also prone to strokes and peripheral vessel, or leg vessel, disease.

LACK OF EXERCISE
In the light of research, which shows that regular exercise improves the circulation and protects the heart, lack of exercise is clearly a risk factor.

With industrialization, automation and mechanized transport, there has been a great decrease in the amount of physical activity in the last few decades. Nowadays, few people are employed in heavy manual jobs. In technologically advanced countries most jobs are light. Leisure time activity is therefore the major source of physical exercise.

In a study of middle-aged civil servants in London, published in 1980, men reporting vigorous leisure time activities had only about one-third the rate of coronary heart disease compared with men of similar age who did not take any vigorous exercise. Examples of vigorous exercise include swimming, "keep fit" exercises, jogging, running, brisk walking, cycling, climbing many stairs, and doing heavy work in the garden, house or garage.

THE CONTRACEPTIVE PILL
Women of 40 to 44 years of age who take the contraceptive pill are five to six times more likely to develop coronary heart disease than their peers who do not take the pill. The link between the contraceptive pill and high blood pressure in susceptible women is discussed in Chapter 7 (see page 70).

Women on the pill are at particularly high risk if they also have other risk factors, such as a raised level of blood lipids or hypertension, or if they smoke cigarettes. If you are over the age of 40, smoke or have a family history of coronary heart disease, you should use an alternative method of contraception.

WATER HARDNESS
Death rates from coronary heart disease in the United Kingdom are higher in soft water areas than hard water areas. The death rate in the south and east of England, for example, where the water is predominantly hard, is low; in the north and west, on the other hand, where the water is softer, the death rate from coronary heart disease is 40 per cent higher. Soft water has a particularly high salt content. It is also more acidic than hard water, so it is likely to dissolve potentially toxic elements, such as lead, cadmium and chromium. There is, however, no evidence that these toxic elements are involved in the increased risk of coronary heart disease. If domestic water softeners are used, it may be worth making sure that they do not affect the drinking water.

5

Stress: a neglected risk factor

Stress is a highly complex and personal matter. It affects all of us in the way we feel, behave, perform at work, and fall prey to accidents or illness. Stress occurs whenever we feel under any pressure. It is also a response to any situation to which we are not accustomed. It is virtually impossible to formulate an accurate definition of stress because it varies so much according to a person's perception of a situation, as well as his ability to cope with it.

THE PERCEPTION OF STRESS

Different people, when confronted with the same information, situation or problem, will respond to it in different ways. What feels like overwhelming stress to one person may be a stimulating challenge to another, or a mere trifle to a third person.

Our genetic endowment, upbringing, education and previous experience in dealing with such situations will determine whether they are challenging, threatening, acceptable or boring and, hence, the response they will produce. This can be subjective, such as feelings of anxiety and tension; physiological, such as a rise in blood pressure; or behavioural, such as drinking too much alcohol or defying authority.

Some stress is necessary

A certain amount of stress is essential for our personal growth: it gives us a zest for life, spurs us on, keeps us going and makes us creative. Too few challenges make our lives boring and frustrating and this can be just as stressful as too many challenges. It has been said that finding the right balance is like adjusting the strings of a musical instrument to obtain a melodious tune: too loose and the tune will be ruined, too tight and the strings will break.

Stress is a fact of life: we can't escape it. Any change, pleasant or not, is stressful to some degree. A new love affair, getting married, going on holiday and being promoted are all examples of a positive kind of stress. Bereavement, being burgled and breaking a leg, on the other hand, are all negative types of stress, but as long as these experiences are few and far between, most of us would recover from them without any long-term ill effects.

Becoming tense over making a difficult decision, getting anxious about the outcome of an uncertain situation, worrying about the problems of relationships with others, and feeling frightened when faced with dangers are all perfectly normal reactions. The stress response prepares us to face all these difficult situations.

Chronic stress

When several stressful things happen all at once, recovery may be slow but it can still occur, providing that we have the necessary coping abilities and stressful situations do not keep repeating themselves. It is only when stress – usually of a subtle kind continuing for a prolonged period – is beyond control and relief that the strain begins to tell. Examples of this kind of chronic stress include:

● Long-standing marital disharmony
● Litigation involving a bitter conflict
● The struggle to keep a business solvent through a recession
● Working under an unpleasant boss or with an incompetent subordinate
● A difficult and persistent conflict of loyalties
● Public disgrace and demotion at work through no fault of your own
● Being made redundant with no prospects of finding a job in the foreseeable future
● The death of a spouse or child.

Circumstances such as these can result in distress or disease. The difficulty is that the victim is not always aware that he is under stress until a crisis occurs. Only when a nervous breakdown or a heart attack occurs does it become easier to look back and understand more clearly.

It is also important to be aware that stress does not only come in large parcels. The little things in everyday living such as driving in a traffic jam,

constant interruption while under sustained pressure to meet repeated deadlines, having to put up with incompetent superiors, not being appreciated for good work or having to wait in all day for a repair man can all build up and take a major toll on your general health.

Susceptibility to stress

When stress is so excessive or prolonged that it becomes a way of life, it can lead to mental, emotional and physical fatigue. And in a susceptible individual, this can result in cardiovascular disease.

Since individuals differ greatly, not only in their genetic susceptibility but also in their perception of stress and their ability to cope, it is impossible to predict precisely the degree of strain or disability that will result from a particular stress. Thus it is difficult to devise experiments to demonstrate the link between stress and heart disease.

There is, on the other hand, a considerable amount of circumstantial evidence which points to stress, resulting from social, psychological, occupational, cultural, personality and behavioural factors, contributing to ill health and death from cardiovascular disease. In a recent survey on heart disease in the United Kingdom several thousand working men were asked what they thought was the most important cause of heart attacks: "stress" was the number one answer.

This was not, however, the first indication that stress might be a contributory factor in heart disease. Since ancient times, as far back as the biblical era, people have always believed stress to be an important factor in diseases of the heart. And in a public survey carried out in the United States in 1973, "emotional pressure, worry and anxiety" were perceived as the most likely causes of high blood pressure.

HOW TO RECOGNIZE STRESS

In order to recognize the signs and symptoms of stress in yourself or anyone else, it is necessary to understand what effect it has on the body and mind and on behaviour.

The "fight or flight" mechanism

Whenever we receive a stress signal, whether real or imaginary, a biological mechanism called the "fight or flight" response comes into operation. The situations that cause this response are known as stressors.

● As soon as the brain receives a stress signal, the production of adrenaline and other stress hormones is stepped up.

● The liver releases sugar and fats, which flow into the bloodstream to provide fuel for quick energy.

● Respiration becomes faster, providing more oxygen, although the oxygen supply may become erratic if the chest muscles are tense.

● Red blood cells flood the bloodstream, carrying more oxygen to the muscles of the limbs and brain.

● The heart beats faster and blood pressure rises, ensuring that sufficient blood reaches the necessary areas. This can sometimes be felt as a pounding heart or racing pulse.

● The blood-clotting mechanism is activated in anticipation of injury. This clotting mechanism ensures that the clots seal up the injured blood vessels.

● The muscles become tense in preparation for action: leg muscles are tense in readiness to run; fists and jaw are clenched, ready to fight.

● Digestion ceases, so blood may be diverted to the muscles and brain.

● Perspiration increases in anticipation of the heat that may be induced by fighting.

● The mouth feels dry.

● The bowel and bladder muscles may become loose so there may be a desire to defecate and/or urinate.

● The pupils dilate to let more light in so that you can see in the dark.

● The senses are heightened, enabling quick action and decision making.

The person who undergoes these changes is in a prime state of readiness to deal with danger, challenge, or other real or imaginary demands. It is also important, however, to recognize that this state is a temporary one, reserved to deal with emergencies. The body cannot maintain it as a lasting condition.

Once the immediate threat has been removed or overcome, or after we have adapted to the disturbance, a reverse mechanism is activated and the body returns to its normal state. If, however, the stressor persists, another stressor develops or the resistance continues after the stressor has been removed, the alarm stage is replaced by a stress response which can show itself in a variety of ways.

Biological effects of stress

Blood pressure may stay up or muscles may remain tense, and health may be temporarily or even permanently damaged. The result may be chest discomfort, overbreathing, a feeling of breathlessness or choking, tremor, palpitation, tension headaches, muscle aches, tiredness, indigestion, diarrhoea, frequent urination, a feeling of faintness and so on. If a doctor were to examine you, he might find that you have high blood pressure.

Psychological effects of stress

The mind's ability to interpret situations provides an infinite variety of ways of reacting to stress. A few of the

more common psychological experiences that can result from prolonged stress, which vary from person to person and from time to time, are:
● Inability to concentrate
● Difficulty in making simple decisions
● Loss of self-confidence
● Irritability or frequent anger
● Worry or anxiety
● Irrational fear or outright panic
● Feelings of depression.

Behavioural effects of stress

Stress may also reveal its presence in a variety of visible changes in behaviour. Everyone has their own idiosyncratic pattern of stress response, so warning signs are varied. They may include:
● An increase in smoking
● Increased use of medication
● Absent-mindedness
● Accident-proneness
● Reckless driving
● Excessive hand and teeth clenching
● Mannerisms such as hair pulling, nail biting, foot tapping
● Increase or decrease in appetite
● Increased or decreased desire to sleep
● Increased use of alcohol or other recreational drugs
● Uncharacteristic aggression, or Type A behaviour (see page 54).

Fixed stress reactions

Many stress reactions become "conditioned" or "fixed". For instance, a child may have a series of unpleasant experiences with people in authority. A fearful reaction whenever he meets such persons becomes habitual. The reaction may be shown in a variety of ways: headaches, stomachache, vomiting, giddiness, a rash or becoming withdrawn.

Years later, the adult may find himself in similar situations which are not really threatening, such as being given a ticket by a policeman. However, the person becomes panic-stricken, starts shaking and displays a habitual pattern of reaction. The reaction is not to the present minor stress, but to the fixed one inside.

How stressed are you?

In order to assess your stress level, answer the stress self-assessment questionnaire opposite.

STRESS AND HEART DISEASE

Many astute physicians of the past have observed relevant and often profound details showing associations between psychological stress and the symptoms of angina or heart attack.

As far back as 1768, an English physician called William Heberden added to his vivid description of angina, ". . . the disease is increased by the disturbance of the mind". John Hunter, a nineteenth-century surgeon from St George's Hospital in London, is reported to have said, "My life is at the mercy of any fool who shall put me in passion!"; he proved his point by dying suddenly during a heated discussion in a boardroom meeting. In 1910, William Osler – in one of his lectures given at the Royal Society of Medicine – said, "a coronary prone man is a keen and ambitious man, the indicator of whose engine is set full speed ahead".

In 1945 the American scientist, Kemple, described a coronary-prone man as "an aggressive, ambitious individual with an intense emotional drive, unable to delegate authority or responsibility with ease, possessing no hobbies and concentrating all his thoughts and energy in the narrow groove of his

STRESS SELF-ASSESSMENT CHART

Rate your status on each item of the following list, with references to the past month. If you have not experienced a particular item at all, score 1; if you have been bothered by it occasionally, score 2; if frequently, score 3; and if daily, score 4.

Cause of stress	Never	Occasionally	Frequently	Almost daily
1 Tension headaches	1	2	3	4
2 Difficulty in falling or staying asleep	1	2	3	4
3 Fatigue	1	2	3	4
4 Overeating	1	2	3	4
5 Constipation	1	2	3	4
6 Lower back pain	1	2	3	4
7 Allergy problems	1	2	3	4
8 Feelings of nervousness	1	2	3	4
9 Nightmares	1	2	3	4
10 High blood pressure	1	2	3	4
11 Hives	1	2	3	4
12 Alcohol consumption	1	2	3	4
13 Minor infections	1	2	3	4
14 Indigestion	1	2	3	4
15 Hyperventilation (rapid breathing)	1	2	3	4
16 Worrisome thoughts	1	2	3	4
17 Treatment for pre-menstrual tension	1	2	3	4
18 Menstrual distress	1	2	3	4
19 Nausea or vomiting	1	2	3	4
20 Irritability with others	1	2	3	4
21 Migraine headaches	1	2	3	4
22 Early morning awakening	1	2	3	4
23 Loss of appetite	1	2	3	4
24 Diarrhoea	1	2	3	4
25 Aching neck and shoulder muscles	1	2	3	4
26 Asthma attack	1	2	3	4
27 Colitis attack	1	2	3	4
28 Periods of depression	1	2	3	4
29 Arthritis pain	1	2	3	4
30 Common cold or 'flu	1	2	3	4
31 Minor accidents	1	2	3	4
32 Tranquillizers or anti-depressants	1	2	3	4
33 Peptic ulcer	1	2	3	4
34 Cold hands or feet	1	2	3	4
35 Heart palpitations	1	2	3	4
36 Sexual problems	1	2	3	4
37 Angry feelings	1	2	3	4
38 Difficulty in communicating with others	1	2	3	4
39 Inability to concentrate	1	2	3	4
40 Difficulty in making decisions	1	2	3	4
41 Feelings of low self-esteem	1	2	3	4
42 Feelings of depression	1	2	3	4

Score analysis

The minimum score for a man is 40 (42 for women) and the maximum score is 160 (168 for women). The higher the score, the more stressed you are. Most people suffer from one or two of these problems. Remember, too, that this score is only for one month.

■ **Under 50:** you are doing very well.
■ **50-80:** you are mildly stressed.
■ **81-109:** you are moderately stressed.
■ **110 or more:** you urgently need to reduce your stress level.

career". While Harold Wolf, another American scientist, described him in 1958 as one "who not only meets challenge by putting out extra effort, but who takes little satisfaction from his accomplishment".

BEHAVIOUR TYPES

Observations such as Kemple's or Wolf's, though pertinent, are not admissible as evidence in medical science. Despite their difficulties, scientific studies into the coronary-prone person have identified a type of behaviour known as Type A which has been accepted, at least in the United States, as one of the major coronary risk factors. The Type A person is described as having an excessive sense of urgency, a preoccupation with deadlines and intense competitiveness.

How this was established

Twenty years ago, two San Francisco cardiologists, Mayer Friedman and Ray Rosenman, called in a furniture upholsterer to repair the furniture in their waiting room. He asked the doctors what kind of patients they treated; when the doctors enquired why he was asking that question, he said, "they all seem to be sitting on the edges." Their interest in the subject kindled by this and other chance observations, Friedman and Rosenman went on to suggest that a certain behaviour pattern might be instrumental in the causation of coronary heart disease. This they called Type A behaviour, as opposed to Type B, which is more relaxed and easy-going.

Type A behaviour

Dr Rosenman says that "a Type A individual is one who is involved in a chronic, excessive struggle to achieve an unlimited number of things in the shortest possible time, perhaps against obstruction by other things or persons. The Type A individual does not despair of losing the struggle, but continuously grapples with an endless succession of challenges. The Type A person attempts to think, perform and communicate all at once and, in general, lives more rapidly than do his peers."

Typical behaviour exhibited by the Type A person includes rapid body movements, explosive speech, exaggerated intonation during conversation, taut facial gestures and excessive hand and teeth clenching. It has been suggested that this type of behaviour is elicited in susceptible individuals by any circumstances where their competence and mastery is threatened.

This is reflected in certain physiological reactions, such as an increase in blood pressure; a greater release of adrenaline and noradrenaline; and an increased stickiness of platelets in the blood, which leads to a greater likelihood of the formation of blood clots in response to challenge. It is interesting to note that, despite hyperactive reaction to challenging circumstances, the average resting blood pressure of a Type A person is no greater than that of a Type B person.

Type A people are unable to tolerate delays and have difficulty in relaxing. They always work at their maximum capacity, even on a seemingly unimportant task. They do not admit defeat or tiredness but tend rather to suppress fatigue and thus continue to perform, despite exhaustion. They are therefore unlikely to be aware of, or unwilling to acknowledge, their exhaustion, which is often a warning sign of an impending heart attack. Studies have shown that Type As are twice as likely to die of heart attacks as Type Bs.

BEHAVIOUR TEST

Answer each question by circling the number on the scale, from 1 to 8, that best applies to your behaviour.

1 Casual about appointments   1   2   3   4   5   6   7   8   Never late

2 Not competitive   1   2   3   4   5   6   7   8   Very competitive

3 Never feel rushed even under pressure   1   2   3   4   5   6   7   8   Always rushed

4 Tackle one thing at a time   1   2   3   4   5   6   7   8   Try to do several things at once

5 Slow in doing things (eating, walking, talking)   1   2   3   4   5   6   7   8   Hurry in everything

6 Think before expressing feelings   1   2   3   4   5   6   7   8   Impulsive in expressing yourself

7 Many interests   1   2   3   4   5   6   7   8   Few interests outside work

Interpretation of scores
Now add up your scores and see into which category you fall.
- **Less than 30:** Definite Type B
- **30-33:** Possible Type B
- **34-36:** Possible Type A
- **37-40:** Moderate Type A
- **Over 40:** Extreme Type A

Type A behaviour is not inherited but the pressures of modern society often bring out the worst in people and make them behave in a Type A manner.

Which type are you?
If you would like to know whether you are a Type A or a Type B person, do the test above. There are, of course, shades of personality, from extreme Type A, through moderate and possible Type A, to possible and definite Type B, all of which this test takes into account. If you are a Type A, don't despair: it is possible to change the way you act and react, see Chapter 14.

FACTORS AFFECTING STRESS LEVEL

Many different factors in environment can contribute to the amount of stress in your life. It can be the result of work problems, where you live and whether you have moved from one environment to another, for example, from the country to the city, the amount of sleep you are getting or the situation at home.

STRESS AT WORK
Workload, stress and pressure of work are all terms that are deeply embedded in the culture of industrialized societies. Despite mechanization and automation, most people seem to be working longer hours. Looking into the background of young patients who have had heart attacks, it was found that they were more likely to be working harder, doing 50 to 60 hours per week and holding two or even three jobs simultaneously, compared with the control group who had not suffered a heart attack.

Any combination of the following may increase the risk of your having a heart attack, particularly if you have no control over your job:
● Work overload

- Periods of unemployment
- Increased job responsibility
- Holding down more than one job
- Too little responsibility
- Understimulation
- Problems with superiors
- Heavy, demanding physical work
- Work pressures due to piecework remuneration.

Loss of prestige at work, lack of recognition or support by superiors, frustration about job status, night shifts, frequent relocation, financial and other professional worries, as well as dissatisfaction with what you do, may also increase your risk of developing coronary heart disease. In general, it is not the objective rating of any particular occupation but the subjective rating of stress which is more important in the development or progression of coronary heart disease.

LACK OF SLEEP

Living in a constant state of stress can lead to exhaustion. Healthy fatigue, resulting from vigorous exercise, for example, which can be remedied by a good night's sleep, is very different from exhaustion, which may result in sleeplessness and inefficiency at work, which in turn cause even greater stress and greater exhaustion. Regular sleep is the best safeguard against stretching yourself to the point of exhaustion, and the quality of sleep is greatly aided by regular physical activity and learning how to relax properly (see Chapters 13 and 14).

A study of 50-year-old men in Sweden showed that those who slept for eight to twelve hours a night had only half the incidence of high blood pressure, compared with those who slept between four and a half to seven hours a night. Night shift workers had a significantly high rate of high blood

pressure and were found to be more likely to have a heart attack.

SOCIO-ECONOMIC FACTORS

Coronary heart disease used to be more common in affluent professional and executive classes, the theory being that they were subject to more occupational strain than the poorer, manual labourer class. Since the Second World War, however, the picture has reversed and the death rate among unskilled workers is now substantially higher compared with executives and administrators. This is in direct contrast with the general pattern, which shows that heart attacks are more common in rich industrialized countries.

In a study involving 18,000 civil servants in London over a period of eight years, published in 1978, it was shown that, compared with administrators, messengers and other unskilled workers had over three times the death rate from coronary heart disease. It has also been shown, in the survey carried out at Framingham in Massachusetts, that the average blood pressure of those with higher education was lower than that of the people who were not as well educated.

Combined with other risk factors

Only part of this excess death rate can be explained by traditional risk factors such as smoking, high blood pressure and obesity. It may also be that modern working practices and current socio-economic conditions are particularly stressful to people in lower socio-economic groups. Moreover, these people are always the last to receive any health education message.

However, this reversal of pattern is not universal. In Northern India, for example, heart attacks are more common in the richer class. In South

Africa, which probably has the highest rate of heart attacks, heart attacks are more common among whites than among blacks. Among African and West Indian immigrants in England and Wales, the death rate from cardio-vascular diseases tends to be higher in those with skilled and non-labouring jobs compared with those in unskilled manual jobs. It may be that an increase in the rate of heart disease is a con-sequence of relatively recent affluence, involving a process of adjustment to changes in environments. As people get used to their new environments, so the risk not only stops increasing but may also start declining. Part of this recent increase in affluence may be associated with an increase in body weight, cigar-ette smoking and blood pressure.

GEOGRAPHICAL MOBILITY

People usually adjust their behaviour according to their perception of the society in which they live. When the social and cultural basis of their society changes because of moving from one geographical area to another, or from one culture to another, people have to adapt to meet the new demands and expectations.

An increase in social and geographical mobility occurred during the process of industrialization that followed the First World War in Britain, the United States and Canada. With the increased mobility came a quadrupling of the death rate from coronary heart disease, which reached its peak in 1960.

In the Soviet Union and Eastern Europe, on the other hand, the death rate from coronary heart disease has risen more recently. It may be that their diets and smoking habits are also chang-ing, but social stress may well account for a large part of the increase in risk. The urbanization and industrialization

which occurred in the Soviet Union between the years 1945 and 1960 accomplished a degree of change that took 50 years or more in most other developed countries. During this period, migration from one area to another reached record figures.

Immigrant communities

Israel, which has a large population of immigrants, has naturally been the subject of research into the effects on health of moving from one culture to another. Although death rates in immi-grants follow much the same pattern as those in the country from which they originally came, there is a general rise in the death rate from heart attacks. The rate continues to rise in the first gener-ation of children born to immigrants, but then begins to subside in the second generation. It is possible that the immigrants have no great difficulties in accepting themselves as foreigners, while their children face problems of identity. They cannot identify them-selves with the true natives of Israel, at the same time they have nothing in common with the country of their parents' origin; by the second gener-ation, identity with Israel is gradually established.

In an American study of 35,000 people whose histories were followed for up to 25 years, the investigators found that fewer American natives, whose lives remained relatively un-changed, had high blood pressure compared with Chinese and Hungarian immigrants, who had been exposed to profound changes in their social and physical environments. Even among American natives with similar occu-pations, the incidence of high blood pressure was greater in people who had less education and who were living away from their families.

Moving from rural areas to cities

The difference in observed blood pressure depends on the way in which man adapts to changing environments. In support of this are some very marked urban-rural differences. More people in cities generally suffer from high blood pressure than those living in rural areas.

In one study, the blood pressure of South African Zulu people living in villages was compared with that of those who had recently moved to cities and of those who had been settled in the cities for many years. The blood pressure of those who had recently moved to the cities was indeed high. When people have to leave their familiar surroundings with unchanged and unchallenged traditions and move to new areas – for instance during war, revolution, slum-clearance, industrialization and urbanization – their blood pressure begins to rise. However, once the process of adaptation is completed, blood pressure may settle down, but once again this may not be until the second or even third generations.

Similarly, population studies have shown that hypertension is relatively rare in primitive societies, compared with more stressful, industrialized environments. The gradual rise in blood pressure with advancing age, so common in the west, is absent in certain communities in Africa and some islands in the Pacific, unless people adopt a Western way of life.

SOCIAL MOBILITY

Just as moving from one geographical area to another puts demands on a person's adaptive behaviour, so does moving from one job to another, and from one socio-economic class to another. Firstly, people have to work much harder to move up than those who are simply born rich or who stay in their own social class. Secondly, they tend to eat more, drink more, smoke more and exercise less as they enjoy their new-found wealth. Thirdly, they often cut themselves off from their own society and their childhood friends from whom they once derived social, emotional and material support in times of need. And finally, in spite of their wealth, they do not always fit easily into the conventions of the higher tier society to which they are trying to belong.

CULTURAL FACTORS

There is some evidence that social and cultural factors may interact with biological risk factors to influence our susceptibility to coronary heart disease. In Japan, the occurrence of this disease is the lowest in the world. When the Japanese move to Hawaii, their likelihood of getting coronary heart disease is increased to an intermediate level; but when they move to California, the likelihood increases still further and resembles the American rate. It has been suggested that the very low incidence of death from coronary heart disease in Japan might be due in part to the support that the Japanese derive from strong family bonds and group cohesiveness.

Dr Michael Marmot and Professor Lennard Syme from the University of Berkeley, California, have demonstrated that those Japanese-Americans who have maintained traditional Japanese ways of life while in California have a lower rate of coronary heart disease compared with Japanese-Americans who have adopted an American way of life. This difference cannot be adequately explained by the difference in traditional risk factors mentioned earlier, such as high blood pressure, cigarette smoking, blood cholesterol level, obesity or diabetes.

STRESS TEST

Which of these changes have occurred in your life in the past year? Add together the point values (Life Change Units, LCU) of these events.

Event	LCU	Event	LCU
Death of a spouse	100	Outstanding personal achievement	28
Marital separation	65	Revision of personal habits	24
Death of a close family member	63	Trouble with business superior	23
Personal injury or illness	53	Change in work hours or conditions	20
Marriage	50	Change in residence	20
Loss of job	47	Change in schools	20
Marital reconciliation	45	Change in recreation	19
Retirement	45	Change in social activities	18
Change in health of a family member	44	Taking out a small mortgage on home	17
Pregnancy	40	Change in sleeping habits	16
Sex difficulties	39	Change in number of family get-togethers	15
Gain of a new family member	39	Change in eating habits	15
Sudden change in financial status	38	Vacation	13
Death of a close friend	37	Minor violations of law	11
Change to a different kind of work	36		
Increase or decrease in rows with partner	35		
Taking out a big mortgage on your home	31	**Interpretation of scores**	
Foreclosure of mortgage or loan	30	Now add up your scores and see into which	
Change in work responsibilities	30	category you fall.	
Son or daughter leaving home	29	■ **0–149:** Low stress	
Trouble with in-laws	29	■ **150–199:** Mild stress	
Spouse beginning or stopping work	29	■ **200–299:** Moderate stress	
		■ **300 or more:** High stress	

STRESSFUL LIFE EVENTS

Folklore abounds with stories describing people whose hearts have stopped in a setting of overwhelming emotional stress. Typical stressors involve an intense sense of threat, danger, loss and, paradoxically, release. The important factor in these situations is that, in most cases, they are unpredictable and are those over which an individual has no control.

When a number of survivors of heart attacks were interviewed within three days of their onset, significantly more patients reported that they had experienced disturbing life events in the weeks before the heart attack compared with healthy subjects. It is difficult to claim that such events actually cause atherosclerosis, for example, although they can precipitate a heart attack in a person who already has diseased coronary arteries, and occasionally in those with healthy coronary arteries.

Death from a broken heart may be a figure of speech from a bygone age, but bereavement does generally take its toll on health. Indeed, a study involving more than 4,000 widowers in Britain in 1956 showed that their death rate was 40 per cent higher than in those who had not been widowed, and heart attacks were by far the most common cause. Other studies have shown similar results in men and women.

Two American doctors, R.H. Rahe and T.H. Holmes, compiled a stress test by asking many people to rate stress for several life situations compared with getting married which was given a score of 50. The results were then computed in "life change units" (LCU) for each situation. Try the test to see how much stress you have in your life.

LINK WITH OTHER RISK FACTORS

As well as precipitating Type A behaviour (see page 54), stress contributes to other risk factors such as, overeating (see page 47), smoking (see page 41), and an increased consumption of alcohol and coffee (see pages 46 to 47).

Smoking

Cigarette smoking has for a long time been known to be a risk factor. There is some evidence that smoking occasional cigarettes may cause arousal but that

heavy smoking may have a calming effect. This may explain why some people smoke more while under stress.

There is no doubt that smokers find it harder to stop smoking when they are under stress. It is not uncommon for people to become very irritable for a period when they do give up.

Obesity

Most obese people acknowledge that they go on a binge when they are under

---

YOUR PERSONAL RISK PROFILE

The following chart will help you calculate your own risk of heart disease.

1 Age — Score
- ☐ Under 20 — 0
- ☐ 20–40 — 1
- ☐ 41–55 — 2
- ☐ Over 55 — 3

2 Sex
- ☐ Male — 1
- ☐ Female — 0

3 Family history
- ☐ No close relative had a stroke or heart attack — 0
- ☐ 1–2 close relatives had a stroke or heart attack over the age of 60 — 1
- ☐ 1–2 close relatives had a stroke or heart attack under the age of 60 — 4
- ☐ Several close relatives had a stroke or heart attack under the age of 60 — 6

4 Personal history
- ☐ No history of angina, stroke or heart attack — 0
- ☐ Angina — 2
- ☐ Heart attack or stroke when over the age of 50 — 4
- ☐ Heart attack or stroke under 50 — 6

5 Social class
- ☐ Professional, executive, administrator — 0
- ☐ Skilled worker — 1
- ☐ Semi-skilled or unskilled worker — 2

6 Diabetes
- ☐ Never had diabetes — 0
- ☐ Diabetes over the age of 40 controlled on diet only — 1
- ☐ Diabetes over the age of 40 controlled on pills — 2

- ☐ Diabetes started under the age of 40 and on insulin — 3

7 High blood pressure — Score
- ☐ Systolic pressure under 120mm of mercury — 0
- ☐ 120–139mm of mercury — 1
- ☐ 140–159mm of mercury — 2
- ☐ 160–199mm of mercury — 3
- ☐ 200–219mm of mercury — 4
- ☐ 230mm and over — 6

If you do not know your blood pressure level but have been told by your doctor that you have:
- ☐ mild hypertension — 3
- ☐ moderately severe hypertension — 6

8 Tobacco smoking
- ☐ Never smoked or have given up cigarette smoking for more than 5 years — 0
- ☐ Pipes and cigars or ex-cigarette smoker under 5 years — 1
- ☐ Fewer than 10 cigarettes a day — 2
- ☐ 11–20 cigarettes a day — 3
- ☐ 21–40 cigarettes a day — 4
- ☐ 41 or more cigarettes a day — 6

9 Blood cholesterol level
- ☐ Under 180mg (less than 4.9mmol/l) — 0
- ☐ 180–218mg (4.9–5.63mmol/l) — 1
- ☐ 218–240mg (5.63–6.20mmol/l) — 2
- ☐ 240–268mg 6.20–6.93mmol/l) — 4
- ☐ More than 268mg (over 6.93mmol/l — 6

---

stress. When they are under pressure, they eat without realising what they are doing until afterwards. Some even claim that they seem to think better when they eat. Stress often drives people to alcohol, too, and alcohol can lead, independently, to both obesity and high blood pressure thus increasing the risks.

Blood lipids

Stress can also contribute to a rise in blood lipids. In a study conducted by Doctors Friedman and Rosenman on a group of accountants in the United States, just before the tax deadline of 15th April, repeated blood tests showed a gradual rise in blood cholesterol, reaching its peak in April, and a rapid decline after the tax deadline. In another study of new cadets admitted to the United States Air Force Academy, cholesterol levels were at their highest during the initial weeks; once the stressful phase of training was over, the cholesterol levels decreased. Cholesterol levels have also been noticed to rise in medical students just before their important final year exams.

	Score
If you do not know the level of your blood cholesterol but have been told that your cholesterol is:	
☐ slightly raised	2
☐ moderately raised	4
☐ high	6

10 Diet (based on consumption of nearly all items listed in each group)

	Score
☐ One or more daily servings of red meat or offal; more than 7 eggs a week; daily consumption of butter and cheese; 300-600ml (½-1 pint) of whole milk; more than 150ml (¼ pint) cream a week	6
☐ Red meat or offal 4-6 times a week; 4-7 eggs a week; 300ml (½ pint) or less milk daily; daily consumption of butter	3
☐ Red meat 3 times or less a week; 2-4 eggs a week, fish, poultry and polyunsaturated margarine; 300ml (½ pint) of skimmed or semi-skimmed milk; cheese or cream 2-3 times a week	2
☐ Fish and poultry; occasional red meat, cheese, cream and butter; 2 or less eggs a week; soft margarine, skimmed milk	1
☐ Vegetarian diet, including yogurt, skimmed milk, cottage cheese, nuts, whole grains, beans, cereals, fruits and vegetables, sunflower or other polyunsaturated oils and soft polyunsaturated margarine	0

11 Stress

	Score
☐ Life feels like a chronic, joyless struggle; feeling of being trapped	4
☐ Chronic struggle; frequently angry, occasionally losing control	3
☐ Repeated challenge; frustrated, bored or under-stimulated	2
☐ Refreshingly challenged, able to rise above the challenges and yet relaxed and easy going. Having a sense of purpose and accomplishment	0

12 Weight

	Score
☐ Less than 4.5kg (10lb) overweight	0
☐ Between 4.5-11.5kg (10-25lb) overweight	2
☐ More than 11.5kg (25 lb) overweight	4

13 Exercise

	Score
☐ Involved in some form of vigorous exercise (cycling, hard swimming, aerobics) 3 times a week or more	0
☐ Reasonably active (regular yoga, leisurely swimming, keep fit exercises, walking etc.)	1
☐ Sedentary, very little exercise (office work, light house work)	3

How to interpret your score

Now add up your scores and see into which category you fall.

- **0-10:** Lower than the average risk
- **11-20:** Average risk
- **21-30:** Moderately high risk
- **31-40:** High risk
- **41-50:** Very high risk
- **More than 50:** Dangerously high risk

6

Atherosclerosis

How do the risk factors discussed in the last two chapters actually increase your risk? The answer to this question, in a nutshell, is by speeding up the process of atherosclerosis.

Derived from the Greek *athere* meaning gruel, and *skleros* meaning hardening, atherosclerosis is the silting up of arteries by deposits of fatty tissue. The effect of this is similar to the build-up of "fur" which clogs the inside of metal pipes, slowing down the flow of water to a trickle so that eventually only drips can come through.

When does atherosclerosis begin?

Streaks of fatty tissue – known as atheroma – are deposited on the inner wall of the arteries from childhood onwards. Indeed, a large majority of the soldiers who died in the Korean war were found to have marked atherosclerosis, yet their average age was 22.

If the lining of the arteries is damaged – as it is thought to be by high blood pressure and cigarette smoking – large patches of fatty deposits are likely to occur over a period of years. These are known as atheromatous plaques and tend to occur at the point where arteries branch (bifurcation), and where the smooth flow of blood is naturally disturbed. Certain arteries are particularly susceptible, including the coronary arteries which supply the heart (as thin as a straw, they are easily blocked); the

carotid arteries in the neck; the cerebral arteries supplying the brain; and the arteries in the legs.

What is the plaque made up of?

Inside the plaque there is a yellow, gruel- or porridge-like substance, which consists mainly of the blood lipids, cholesterol and triglycerides. These lipids are found in the bloodstream, combined with specific proteins to form particles known as lipoproteins. All lipoprotein particles contain cholesterol, triglycerides, phospholipids and protein, but in different proportions.

Lipoproteins all vary in size

Chylomicra are the largest and consist almost entirely of triglycerides. The next in size are the pre-beta lipoproteins, and then the beta lipoproteins, in which the cholesterol component is gradually increased and the triglycerides decreased. Pre-beta and beta lipoproteins are also known as low density and very low density lipoproteins (LDL and VLDL) and are the most significant particles in the development of atheroma. The smallest lipoproteins are the alpha lipoproteins, which contain less cholesterol and triglycerides, and are very rich in proteins. These are known as high density lipoproteins (HDL) and are thought to be protective against the development of atheromatous plaque.

THE LINK BETWEEN LIPOPROTEINS AND ATHEROMA

The theory is that lipoproteins pass between the lining cells of the arteries and some of them accumulate underneath. The only exceptions are the chylomicra, which are too big to pass through. Enzymes present in the wall break down the protein in the lipoproteins leaving the insoluble cholesterol and triglycerides in the elastic layer of the artery. These fats are then trapped and set up a small inflammatory reaction. The alpha particles do not react with the enzymes and are returned to the circulation.

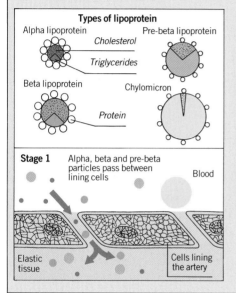

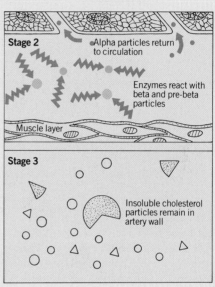

WHAT CAN HAPPEN

The repeated inflammatory reactions caused by lipoproteins becoming trapped in the wall of the artery (see above), cause scarring and the artery walls gradually become hardened. Occasionally, bleeding occurs into the plaques and the artery walls become distorted. Calcium is deposited, rendering the plaque more brittle and liable to crack. The combination of all these processes causes the lining surface layer to break down, producing an ulcer. High blood pressure accelerates the damage by putting greater strain on the already weakened arterial wall.

Various constituents of the blood, such as the red blood cells, platelets, lipids and fibrin (shreds of protein that help to trap the cells), may stick to the raw surface of the plaques. These sticky patches later become fibrous and are eventually incorporated into the artery wall. Thus the plaques will increase in size over the years. If the area is extensive, it progressively reduces the internal diameter of the artery until it becomes very narrow (stenosis). The gradual hardening of the artery (arteriosclerosis) which tends to occur with age further contributes to atherosclerosis.

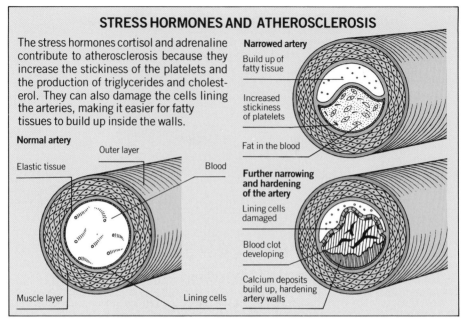

STRESS HORMONES AND ATHEROSCLEROSIS

The stress hormones cortisol and adrenaline contribute to atherosclerosis because they increase the stickiness of the platelets and the production of triglycerides and cholesterol. They can also damage the cells lining the arteries, making it easier for fatty tissues to build up inside the walls.

Narrowed artery
Build up of fatty tissue

Increased stickiness of platelets

Fat in the blood

Normal artery
Outer layer
Elastic tissue
Blood

Further narrowing and hardening of the artery
Lining cells damaged

Blood clot developing

Calcium deposits build up, hardening artery walls

Muscle layer
Lining cells

In about a third of those people who have angina, or who have a heart attack, there is no evidence of atherosclerosis. Coronary artery spasm (sudden temporary constriction of the artery, caused by muscle contraction, see page 83) may be the cause. Nobody knows why a spasm occurs, but stress is one of the suspected factors. Equally, atherosclerosis may be present for years without any indication whatsoever until its first manifestation is a heart attack or a stroke.

Angina

The most common symptom of atherosclerosis is angina – a pain in the chest which occurs when narrowed arteries cannot supply enough oxygen and fuel during exercise and stress. Angina is covered in detail in Chapter 8.

Heart attack or stroke

The raw surface of the plaques of atheroma often increases turbulence in the flow of blood, which may trigger off

the blood's clotting mechanism. Unfortunately, however, clotting inside a damaged but intact artery results in thrombosis. The release of certain hormones during stress, for instance, adrenaline and cortisol, leads to further damage to the artery walls, increases the stickiness of the platelets, and attracts more fatty deposits both in and on the lining of the artery walls.

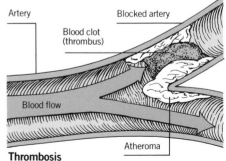

Artery
Blocked artery
Blood clot (thrombus)
Blood flow
Atheroma

Thrombosis
When blood flow in an area is disturbed by the presence of atheromatous plaque, blood cells, particularly platelets, can stick together forming a clot, or thrombus, blocking the artery.

The clot, or thrombus, if it is not dissolved quickly enough, will cut off the blood supply to the area beyond it altogether and part of the organs or tissue supplied by that artery will die. A thrombosis in a coronary artery will lead to a *heart attack* (see Chapter 9). If the artery that is blocked is a relatively large one, like the left main coronary artery, death may be instant. A thrombus or clot in one of the cerebral arteries cuts off blood supply to the brain and causes a *stroke* (see page 24).

Other complications

A minute fragment of atheromatous plaque (embolus) sometimes breaks off and travels free in the circulation, and symptoms depend on which part of the body is being deprived of blood. If an embolus lodges in a small vessel of the brain, then a mini-stroke or transient ischaemic attack may occur. Ischaemia is a condition in which there is an inadequate supply of oxygen. However, in a "transient" attack, the stroke-like symptoms last for only a short time; small emboli and blood clots dissolve by themselves and complete recovery can occur in hours or even minutes. But if the embolus is large, or it occurs repeatedly, it could cause a stroke.

Other possible problems include peripheral vessel disease and kidney damage, which eventually leads to kidney failure. Atherosclerosis can also exacerbate high blood pressure.

If you have chest pains, pains in the calf muscles during exercise or when walking uphill, or if you suddenly experience transient weakness in the muscles of your arm or leg and/or temporary speech disturbance, you must consult your doctor immediately.

TESTS FOR ATHEROSCLEROSIS

There are no simple tests which can detect a modest amount of atherosclerosis, and by the time symptoms occur or an electrocardiogram (see page 37) becomes positive, the process has already advanced considerably. Recent research suggests that, while it may be possible to cause a fatty streak on the lining of an artery to disappear, nothing can be done to reduce an established plaque. Atherosclerosis must therefore be prevented, and if it has already started, its progress must be halted.

It is possible to have atherosclerosis even though you have been told previously that your blood pressure and blood cholesterol level are normal and you do not smoke. As I have already said, there is no absolute cut-off point beyond which blood pressure or the blood cholesterol level becomes "abnormal". The risk of atherosclerosis increases throughout – and even within – the normal range: quite simply, the lower the level, the lesser the risk. Since the risk of developing atherosclerosis is related to the level of cholesterol in your blood, it is very important to eat sensibly. You should also give up cigarettes if you are a smoker, and follow a programme of regular physical activity, which is also believed to impede the development of atherosclerosis. All these subjects are covered in greater detail in Chapters 10, 12 and 14, of the self-help section.

There is no doubt that atherosclerosis runs in families, and that men are more likely to be affected than women, so if a close relative has suffered from atherosclerosis or any other heart disease, you should be particularly careful.

7
High blood pressure

When you are active, excited or under stress, your blood pressure goes up as a matter of course. This rise is essential because exercise and emotions demand extra energy and oxygen, which are provided by an extra supply of blood, delivered under raised pressure (see "fight or flight" mechanism, page 51). Once the activity subsides and you relax, the blood pressure returns to normal. This transient rise is perfectly normal, but if your blood pressure goes up and stays up, even when you are relaxed, you would be said to have high blood pressure, or hypertension.

It must be emphasized here that there is no definitive dividing line between "normal" and "high" blood pressure, in much the same way as there is no clear division between a person of "normal" height and one who is tall. It is not strictly correct, therefore, to talk about individuals as "having" or "not having" high blood pressure. However, despite the reservations about defining normal and high blood pressure, it is obviously convenient to use some such values, arbitrary though these may be.

Definition of high blood pressure
The World Health Organization (WHO) has defined the normal range of blood

pressure as a systolic pressure of 100-140mmHg, and a diastolic pressure of 60-90mmHg. High blood pressure is defined by the WHO as consistently exceeding 160/95mmHg when resting. Blood pressure between 140-160mmHg systolic and 90-95mmHg diastolic is known as borderline hypertension. The severity of high blood pressure is often graded according to the diastolic value alone. Thus when diastolic blood pressure is between 95-105mmHg it is known as mild hypertension; between 105-120mmHg is considered moderately severe; and above that is severe.

Although mild hypertension is, of course, higher than desirable, it probably does not need any drug treatment, at least for people over 65 years of age provided they do not have any other symptoms. In younger people, however, it is preferable to lower it. At all ages, the lower the pressure the better.

Recent population studies suggest that the level of systolic pressure may be as good – if not better – a predictor of the risk of your developing coronary heart disease. The risk increases over the whole range of readings. It has been calculated that in men in their forties, for example, every 10mmHg systolic pressure increases the risk by 20 per cent. Thus a person whose systolic pressure is 160mmHg has twice the risk of a person whose systolic pressure is at 110mmHg; beyond 180mmHg, the rise in risk becomes steeper.

The systolic and diastolic pressures tend to rise together, but this is not necessarily so and some people, particularly the elderly, have a much greater increase in the systolic than in the diastolic pressure; their diastolic pressure may be normal, or near normal.

Are there any obvious symptoms?

Raised blood pressure does not produce any symptoms in the early stages. Many people are under the impression that headaches, particularly early-morning ones, dizziness, nose-bleeds, high-coloured cheeks, heart palpitations and noises in the ears are all symptoms of high blood pressure. These symptoms can, however, be present in people with normal blood pressure and quite high pressure may be present without them.

The only way you can be sure is to have your blood pressure measured. Everyone should have their blood pressure checked every five years and if it is on the higher side of normal, it should be measured more frequently. In fact many general practitioners are measuring the blood pressure of everyone who consults them.

If hypertension is well advanced or has been present for many years, it may cause severe headaches, shortness of breath, giddiness, visual disturbances and disrupted sleep. Hypertension may even present itself for the first time as a sudden crisis: angina, a heart attack, a stroke and various other complications.

How common is it?

High blood pressure is a very common condition in developed countries. It affects approximately 15-30 per cent of middle-aged European men. In Britain, it is estimated that approximately a fifth of the adult population has high blood pressure; relatively fewer younger people have it but one person in five develops it over the age of 40, and the proportion increases still further with advancing age. In the United States, approximately 20 per cent of white men under the age of 30, rising to 35 per cent in those over 55, have been shown to have hypertension. The figures in other industrialized countries are comparable.

What can high blood pressure do?

High blood pressure puts considerable strain on the heart and blood vessels. As a result, the blood vessels become thicker and more rigid. It also accelerates the process of atherosclerosis which, in turn, further contributes to the rise in pressure. The argument is like that of the chicken and the egg: which comes first, atherosclerosis or high blood pressure?

An examination of insurance company records dating from 1915 to 1954 of some five million people (in other words before the introduction of drug treatment for high blood pressure) revealed that even a modest rise in blood pressure was associated with increased chances of early death. For example, healthy men with a blood pressure of 140/90 were found to have one and a half times the chances of dying before the average lifespan of all insured lives. Those with pressures of 145/95 had double the chances of dying early; and those with pressures of 160/100 had three times the chances. To put it another way, a man of 35 years of age with a blood pressure of 150/100 could expect to live 16 years less than his counterpart with a pressure of 120/80.

As I explained earlier, there is no precise cut-off point or critical level of

67

blood pressure beyond which it becomes hypertension and therefore dangerous. The degree of risk is directly related to the height of blood pressure (see page 42). The shortening of life is due to one of the complications outlined in Chapter 2 (see pages 20 to 29). The case histories below serve to illustrate the sort of complications that can result from raised blood pressure.

In a large-scale population study of high blood pressure at Framingham in Massachusetts, 10,000 men and women of 30 to 59 years of age were examined in 1949 and then regularly followed up for 20 years. Those with hypertension – defined as a blood pressure of 160/95 or more – were found to be seven times more prone to strokes, four times more prone to congestive heart failure, and

CASE HISTORIES

Heart attack

John was a messenger in a bank. He liked his food and cigarettes and his lunchtime drinks with friends. One lunchtime he suddenly realized that it was past 2 o'clock and he had to convey important documents to other branches of the bank within the next half hour, so he was a bit pushed for time.

While walking briskly, he felt an ache in his chest. He thought it must be indigestion and would take something for it when he got back, but the ache turned into a vice-like grip. The pain also radiated up into his neck and down his left arm. "What a nuisance," he thought. Maybe he should take the afternoon off but he had to deliver those documents that day and he continued to walk. The next thing he knew, he was in a coronary care unit.

Stroke

Mary was a housewife with a mentally handicapped daughter. She never went to doctors with what seemed to her to be trivial complaints, such as headaches, even occasional slurring of speech or blurring of vision. She always thought that she could not afford to become ill when she had a daughter to take care of. One day she dropped a plate, and for the rest of the day that hand felt useless. The neighbours thought she should see her doctor but Mary wouldn't listen. The next day she woke up with the whole of her right side paralysed and she couldn't get the words out of her mouth. She was admitted to hospital and diagnosed as having had a stroke.

Peripheral vessel disease

Peter always walked to work, but he had begun to find that he had to stop every few hundred metres because of pain in his right calf. Once he stood still, the pain disappeared in a few minutes. The distance he could walk without getting pain was growing shorter and shorter.

Finally, he decided to consult his doctor, he was diagnosed as having "intermittent claudication", from the Latin word for limp, or leg vessel disease. He was advised to stop smoking immediately, some tests were ordered, dietary advice was given and some pills were prescribed. He found it particularly hard to stop smoking and the six to eight pills he was asked to take daily made his life a misery because of their unpleasant side-effects.

Hypertensive encephalopathy

Margaret was 25 with two young children. The couple thought that their family was complete and she was quite happy to be on the contraceptive pill. She led a very active life, working as a full-time teacher. She started having headaches, her vision began to deteriorate, and at times she felt sick. She put it down to too much stress. Her husband forced her to take a rest, but her vision deteriorated further and one day she became drowsy.

In the end, her husband asked for a doctor's visit. The doctor immediately stopped her pills and urgently referred her to a hospital specialist, who diagnosed her condition as hypertensive encephalopathy.

three times more prone to heart attacks, and they had twice the risk of developing peripheral vessel disease.

Parts of the body affected

Hypertension can affect almost any organ in the body, the most important being the brain, heart, kidneys and eyes, and the peripheral blood vessels (in the limbs).

The likelihood of a complication developing depends on how high the blood pressure is, how long it has been high, the rate at which it is rising, the presence or absence of other risk factors, and how the condition is managed. Since the advent of drug treatment for high blood pressure in the early

1950s and the continuous improvement in the new drugs developed, there has been a significant reduction in strokes, heart failure and kidney failure. Unfortunately, the reduction in coronary artery disease is not as impressive.

Doctors agree that the risk of any complication, including heart attacks, can be drastically reduced both by preventive measures and by proper management, which entails not only drug treatment but also several simple self-help measures (see page 77). Since behaviour and lifestyle contribute a great deal to these complications, it is very important, in these preventive measures, to seek early medical advice and to comply with the treatment.

WHAT CAUSES HYPERTENSION?

In about 85 to 90 per cent of all cases of hypertension, no specific organic cause can be found. This is known as essential, or primary, hypertension.

In the remaining 10 to 15 per cent, hypertension is secondary to kidney disease; congenital malformation of the blood vessels; tumours causing secretion of certain hormones; drugs, including the contraceptive pill; and toxaemia of pregnancy.

ESSENTIAL HYPERTENSION

Nobody really knows for certain what causes essential hypertension. It is generally agreed, however, that hypertension occurs as a result of interaction between the hereditary and environmental factors listed right. These are discussed in detail in Chapters 4 and 5. There are a number of risk factors: age, sex and heredity; psychological, social and occupational stress; excessive salt intake, excess alcohol and coffee; obesity; and a sedentary lifestyle.

Even the number of children in the family seems to have some bearing on hypertension In general, the larger the family, the lower the blood pressure in the parents, though why this should be so remains a complete mystery. In some individuals the hereditary factor seems strong, while in others the influence of environmental factors is the stronger component. It is unlikely that any single factor will turn out to be the sole cause of hypertension.

RISK FACTORS FOR ESSENTIAL HYPERTENSION

- Age
- Gender
- Family history
- Race
- Stress:
  psychological
  social
  occupational
- Social class
- Excess alcohol
- Excess coffee
- Smoking
- Diet
- Excess salt and/or too little potassium
- Fat
- Sugar
- Obesity
- Sedentary lifestyle
- Lack of sleep

69

SECONDARY HYPERTENSION

In secondary hypertension, a chronic rise in blood pressure occurs which is secondary to another condition: it can happen when kidneys are extensively damaged – by an inflammatory disease or a tumour, for example – or when blood flow to the kidneys is obstructed. In only a small proportion of these cases, however, is surgery necessary to reverse the condition. In the rest, the management of high blood pressure is the same as in essential hypertension.

Pregnancy

A rise in blood pressure after the 20th week of pregnancy is one of the signs of a complication known as pre-eclamptic toxaemia, or pre-eclampsia. No definite cause for this is known. In addition to the rise in blood pressure, there may also be a protein leak in the urine (which indicates possible kidney damage) and swelling of the ankles as a result of fluid retention.

Once you have developed raised blood pressure, you may need to be admitted to hospital for bed rest. If this does not lower blood pressure, drugs must be given to reduce it, otherwise blood pressure can rise very rapidly leading to fits which may endanger the lives of both you and, especially, your unborn baby. Relaxation in the early stages of pregnancy had been shown to reduce the chances of high blood pressure developing and therefore to reduce the chances of having to be admitted to hospital.

Contraceptive pills

Most contraceptive pills contain a combination of oestrogen and progestogen in varying proportions and may interfere with the renin-angiotensin system, which is involved in regulating the fluid balance in the body. This can cause a slight rise in blood pressure through the retention of salt and water.

A few women, however, are particularly sensitive to the contraceptive pill and develop hypertension. Since the number of women taking the pill is very high, oral contraception probably causes more hypertension than all other recognized causes of secondary hypertension put together. If you are on the pill, you should have your blood pressure checked regularly and, if it rises significantly, you should use an alternative method of contraception. Contraceptive pills also increase the risk of having a heart attack, especially in women over 35 who smoke.

Check with your doctor or family planning clinic that you are on a low-dose pill. It is important that low-dose pills should be prescribed unless there is a special reason, for example, heavy periods, and that you have a break of two or three months every four years. Smokers over 35 years of age should use alternative forms of contraception – such as barrier methods or the coil.

Drugs

Some drugs which are used for depression can cause hypertension if proper dietary advice is not carefully adhered to. In addition, some prescription antibiotics and certain cold remedies and nose drops bought over the counter can also raise blood pressure temporarily by constricting the blood vessels.

Problems with glands

Tumours in the adrenal glands, above the kidneys, or in the pituitary gland, in the brain, also cause hypertension as a result of the excessive secretion of the hormones produced by the affected glands. These hormones include adrenaline, noradrenaline, cortisol, aldosterone, renin, and serotonin. Such cases are extremely rare and are usually diagnosed by specific symptoms and special tests. Successful treatment is usually surgical.

Lead and cadmium poisoning

It is thought that lead and cadmium poisoning may, very rarely, cause hypertension, although the evidence is conflicting. Lead can enter the body through drinking water and the air you breathe, while cadmium is present at very low levels in a variety of foods, especially kidneys, and in some crops and seafoods contaminated by local industrial pollution.

Blood vessel malformation

In one type of congenital malformation the child is born with a constriction in the aorta – the main blood vessel arising from the heart (see page 13) – just beyond the origins of the blood vessels that supply the arms, neck and head. This causes blood pressure to be high in the arms and relatively low in the legs. It can easily be recognized by a doctor, and if corrected surgically, high blood pressure can be completely cured.

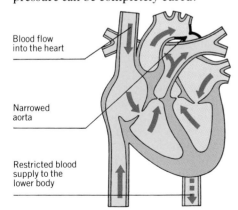

Blood flow into the heart

Narrowed aorta

Restricted blood supply to the lower body

Malformation of aorta
Also known as coarctation of the aorta, this is a localized narrowing of the aorta that reduces the blood supply to the lower part of the body.

SUMMARY OF CAUSES OF SECONDARY HYPERTENSION

- Kidney disease
- Pre-eclamptic toxaemia
- The contraceptive pill and other drugs
- Growths in hormone-secreting glands
- Lead and cadmium poisoning
- Congenital malformation of certain blood vessels.

HOW A TEMPORARY RISE BECOMES PERMANENT

Whatever the causative factors, blood pressure usually rises gradually. In the beginning, it is sometimes up and sometimes down, but it gradually remains higher and higher. The level is usually lower while you are asleep.

Frequent rises in blood pressure mean that the baroreceptors in the artery walls (see page 18) are reset at a higher level so that they no longer recognize higher pressure levels as "high". Once they are reset, they try to maintain the blood pressure within the new higher range.

Frequent rises in blood pressure also cause structural changes in medium-sized, muscular arteries. All muscles develop with use; high blood pressure causes the artery walls to become thicker and more muscular so that they can resist high pressure in the system. The result is that whenever these vessels constrict – for example, in response to stress – the narrowing of the vessels is therefore that much greater and the rise in your blood pressure correspondingly higher.

Eventually, these structural changes not only help to maintain a higher pressure, but also perpetuate it. Thus, it is possible that high blood pressure, once established, could be maintained by a different set of factors from those that initiated it.

DRUG TREATMENT

Drugs are prescribed if hypertension is not satisfactorily controlled by the non-drug measures outlined in the self-help section (see pages 124 to 186). If blood pressure is very high, drug treatment may be started straight away and continued along with other measures. If there is a dramatic response to the combined effort, the quantity of drugs may be reduced. Although different drugs may have to be tried before your blood pressure is successfully controlled, once you start drug treatment, you will probably remain on drugs for the rest of your life. The decision to start drug treatment is therefore an extremely important one. If your doctor comments happily that "your blood pressure is now fine", it does not necessarily mean that you can come off drugs. Please do not stop taking your drugs unless you are specifically told to do so.

THE DO'S AND DON'TS OF DRUG TREATMENT

Do
- Take your pills as prescribed
- Report any side-effects to your doctor
- Have your blood pressure checked regularly
- Take enough pills with you when you are travelling.

Don't
- Forget to take your pills
- Run out of pills
- Start any other medication (including cold remedies) without consulting your doctor
- Miss appointments with your doctor
- Stop taking your medication if you experience side-effects without first consulting your doctor — remember, you can always ring him and describe your side-effects if you are worried.

During the initial stage of adjusting your drug treatment, your doctor will probably want to check your blood pressure frequently – perhaps every one to four weeks. Once your blood pressure is under control, it is usual to measure it every three to six months – your doctor will advise you.

There are four main categories of drug: diuretics, beta-blockers, vasodilators and those that act on the nervous system. Most patients find that diuretics and beta-blockers are effective, either alone or combined.

If you develop any side-effects, do not hesitate to discuss them with your doctor. There is a good chance that a more suitable alternative can be prescribed, and serious side-effects are now, happily, uncommon.

DIURETICS

These are commonly used to start the treatment, although more and more doctors are now using beta-blocking drugs (see page 74) as the first choice.

Diuretics lower blood pressure by reducing the volume of fluid in the circulation. This is done by increasing the amount of salt and water that is excreted by the kidneys, which means that the amount of urine you pass daily will increase, at least to begin with. The cells of the blood vessel walls also lose a certain amount of salt and water and thus become less stiff and less resistant to the blood.

Mild-to-moderate hypertension can often be controlled by diuretics alone. If it is not satisfactorily controlled, beta-blockers are usually added.

Side-effects

Diuretics may have some undesirable side-effects. Although patients do not usually continue to pass large amounts of urine after a few days of treatment, several of the stronger diuretics may continue to have a particularly drastic effect in the first three to four hours after taking them, and this can be both inconvenient and uncomfortable, particularly if you are going out. They can raise the blood sugar level and, in a susceptible person, may precipitate diabetes. People who already have diabetes are not generally prescribed diuretics. These can also raise the blood cholesterol level and some of their beneficial effect may thus be counteracted. They can raise the uric acid level of the blood, which may, on very rare occasions, precipitate an attack of gout. If you already have gout, you should not be treated with diuretics.

Due to their action on the kidneys, diuretics tend to cause some loss of potassium, which is essential for the proper functioning of the body and may even help to bring blood pressure down. Doctors often guard against potassium loss by prescribing pills which combine a diuretic with potassium (indicated by the letter K, which is the chemical symbol for potassium, in the brand name). Some diuretics have a selective action and get rid of sodium, but not potassium; these are known as potassium-sparing diuretics. Most fresh fruits and many vegetables, particularly bananas, grapefruit, oranges, potatoes, and cabbage, are rich in potassium. If you are on diuretics, it is a good idea to include plenty of these in your diet.

Some people are extremely sensitive to diuretics and may lose excessive fluid, which can lead to symptoms such as dizziness, dryness of the mouth, muscle weakness and constipation. Occasionally there may be vomiting, which can make the dehydration even worse. Skin rashes and other allergic

DIURETICS USED TO LOWER BLOOD PRESSURE

Generic name	Trade example	Combined with potassium
bendrofluazide	Centyl	Centyl K
chlorothiazide	Saluric	Saluric K
chlorthalidone	Hygroton	Hygroton K
cyclopenthiazide	Navidrex	Navidrex K
hydrochlorothiazide	Esidrex	Esidrex K
methylchlorothiazide	Enduron	—
polythiazide	Nephril	—
frusemide	Lasix	Lasikal
bumetanide	Burinex	Burinex K
ethacrynic acid*	Edecrin	—
amiloride*	Midamore	Moduretic†
spironolactone*	Aldactone	Aldectide†
triamterene*	Dytac	Diazide†
indapamide	Natrilix **	—
* potassium-sparing	** non-thiazide indoline	† combined with thiazide

reactions may also occur. In a recent large study which was carried out by the Medical Research Council in the United Kingdom, one man in five taking diuretics experienced impotence. However, the diuretic may not be the sole cause of this impotence because atherosclerosis itself can sometimes cause impotence. If the impotence is caused by the diuretic, it will be reversed by stopping the drug.

BETA-BLOCKERS

These drugs can block the effects of the stress hormones adrenaline and norad-renaline at sites called beta receptors in the heart and blood vessels. Other sites affected by these hormones are known as alpha receptors. Foremost among the effects of adrenaline and noradrenaline is that they increase both blood pressure and heart rate. Beta-blockers are particularly useful in dealing with angina, high blood pressure and palpi-tations. They reduce the strain on the heart, by cutting its oxygen demand and reducing the force and speed of the heart beat. However, they also constrict the peripheral blood vessels.

Side-effects

If the heart is already strained by heart disease, then a further reduction in the pumping action of the heart may drive it to failure. If you are already suffering from heart failure, with symptoms such as breathlessness and swollen ankles, you should not be given beta-blockers until the heart failure is under control (see page 24). Similarly, beta-blockers should not be given to anyone whose heart is beating very slowly (a condition known as heart block). One beneficial effect of adrenaline is that it helps to keep the air passages relaxed and open. In susceptible individuals, beta-blockers can lead to wheezing, and are therefore not suitable for asthmatics. One of the

BETA-BLOCKERS USED TO LOWER BLOOD PRESSURE

Generic name	Trade example	Slow-acting preparation	Combined with diuretics
propanolol	Inderal, Angilol, Apsolol, Bedranol, Berkolol	Inderal LA	Inderax, Inderetic
oxprenolol	Trasicor, Loracor, Apsolox	Slow Trasicor Slowpren	Trasidrex
atenolol	Tenormin, Kalten	—	Tenoretic
metoprolol	Lopressor, Betaloc	Betaloc SA	Lopressoretic co-betaloc
acebutolol	Sectral	—	Secadrex
pindolol	Visken, Viskaldix	—	—
timolol	Betim, Prestim Blocadren	—	Moducren
sotalol	Sotacor, Betacardon	—	Sotazide
nadolol	Corgard	—	Corgeretic
betaxolol	Kerlone	—	—
lebetalol*	Trandate, Labrocol	—	—

* beta- and alpha-blocker

most common side-effects of beta-blockers is that the hands and feet get cold because the peripheral vessels become constricted. For this reason, you should not be given beta-blockers if you have leg vessel disease.

Beta-blockers sometimes pass into the brain fluids and can then be responsible for vivid dreams, sleep disturbances and sometimes depression. Patients on beta-blockers commonly complain of feeling tired and not being able to carry out any physical tasks as well as before. There is also a possibility of skin rashes and dry eyes; these should be reported to the doctor who, depending on the severity, may stop the drug. Some beta-blockers raise the level of blood cholesterol and triglycerides (see page 62).

On the whole, however, beta-blockers represent a real advance in the development of drugs for hypertension and are relatively free of side-effects. Most of them have to be taken only once a day, which is also convenient.

Recently, alpha-blockers and drugs which block both beta and alpha receptors have been introduced. They do not constrict the blood vessels, and consequently are preferable to beta-blockers in many cases.

VASODILATORS

A combination of diuretics and beta-blockers is effective in the majority of people with hypertension, but it does not always work. For these patients, the addition of vasodilators is the next logical step. Vasodilators dilate the blood vessels and thus reduce the resistance to the flow of blood in them. They counteract the constriction of blood vessels caused by beta-blockers.

Side-effects

Headaches, palpitations and fluid retention are common side-effects. In

COMMONLY USED VASODILATORS

Generic name	Trade example
hydralazine	Apresoline
prazosin*	Hypovase
minoxidil	Loniten

* also an alpha-blocker

high doses (more than 100mg a day), hydralazine may occasionally give rise to "lupus" syndrome, which can cause a facial rash and arthritic joints, and can damage the kidneys and blood vessels. Prazosin must be started with a very small dose because occasionally, in a sensitive individual, it can lead to an excessive fall in blood pressure and even fainting after the first dose. Minoxidil may stimulate hair growth on the face and body. The discovery of this side-effect has led to the use of minoxidil in alopecia, which causes patchy baldness.

DRUGS ACTING ON THE NERVOUS SYSTEM

These drugs control high blood pressure by interfering with the way in which the brain controls blood pressure.

Methyldopa, reserpine and clonidine are centrally acting, which means they act mainly on the brain itself. Guanethidine, bethanidine and debrisoquine on the other hand, are peripherally acting, which means they block the activity of the nerves that supply the blood vessels.

Side-effects

Most of the centrally acting drugs give rise to depression, fatigue, drowsiness, sleep disturbances and a dry mouth. Methyldopa, as well as guanethidine and bethanidine, commonly produces an excessive fall in blood pressure and dizziness when the patient stands up. If you are taking one of these drugs, avoid standing up too abruptly, and when you get out of bed in the morning, try sitting on the edge of the bed for a few minutes before you stand up. Methyldopa sometimes causes impotence, anaemia or liver damage. Peripherally acting drugs can also produce troublesome diarrhoea and, in men, they can cause impotence and failure to ejaculate.

The majority of these drugs are older generation drugs and their side-effects are both common and relatively more unpleasant than more recent drugs. They are no longer used as drugs of first choice, but they sometimes have to be used if other drugs are for any reason contraindicated, or if blood pressure fails to be controlled by them.

DRUGS ACTING ON THE NERVOUS SYSTEM

	Generic name	Trade example	Combined with diuretics
Centrally acting	reserpine	Serpasil	Rauwiloid Rautrex Serpasil esidrex
	methyldopa	Aldomet, Dopamet, Medomet	Hydromet
	clonidine	Dixarit	Catapres
Peripherally acting	guanethidine	Ismelin	—
	bethanidine	Estbatal, Bendogen	—
	debrisoquine	Declinex	—

CALCIUM ANTAGONISTS

These were originally developed to prevent attacks of angina – and are therefore dealt with in Chapter 8 – but they can also be used to lower blood pressure. They work largely by mopping up the calcium in the artery walls. The arteries then become relaxed and dilated, so reducing the resistance to blood flow, allowing more blood and oxygen to reach the heart muscle. They also help the heart to use oxygen and nutrients more efficiently.

Side-effects

Approximately 40 per cent of those on calcium antagonists complain of side-effects including dizziness and fluid retention, which may be responsible for swollen ankles. Verapamil may cause constipation and rhythm disturbances. But, only five per cent are taken off their drugs on account of their side-effects.

CALCIUM ANTAGONISTS

Generic name	Trade example
diltiazem	Tildiem
nifedipine	Adalat
verapamil	Cordilox

NEW ANTI-HYPERTENSIVES

Captopril (brand names Capoten and Acepril) and enalapril (Innovace) have recently been introduced in the treatment of hypertension. They are known as ACE (which stands for angiotensin converting enzyme) inhibitors because they work by preventing production of a chemical in the blood called angiotensin II, which has a powerful constricting effect on the blood vessels. When angiotensin levels are lowered, the peripheral blood vessels relax and the pressure falls.

Side-effects

There is some evidence that these drugs can impair the action of the kidneys or cause excess fluid loss, which may lead to general weakness and possibly fainting. Occasionally, they have been found to depress the action of the immune system and the formation of blood cells. As with all these drugs, however, it is important that you do not stop taking them without first consulting your doctor, whatever the side-effects.

SELF-HELP

High blood pressure must, if possible, be prevented. If it has already occurred, it must be efficiently controlled to prevent it from advancing further. This is not simply a question of relying on hypertensive drugs: there are a number of ways in which you can help yourself.

If you have been told that you have hypertension, the first and most important thing you can do, if you are a smoker, is to stop smoking (see Chapter 12). And if you are overweight, try to lose weight so as to achieve as near your ideal weight as possible (see page 133).

Changing your diet

What you eat also matters, and eating your way to a healthy heart is discussed in detail in Chapter 10. We all eat far more salt than we actually need, for example, but if you have hypertension it is particularly beneficial to cut down your salt intake. Salt occurs naturally in many foods, so there is no need to add any extra. For a start, don't sprinkle salt over your food at the table, then stop using it in cooking. Cut down on all salty processed foods such as bacon, ham, cheese, smoked fish, salted nuts, crisps and pickles.

Eat fewer animal fats such as butter, cream, cheese, fatty meats and eggs. Eat more wholegrain cereals and pulses, and potassium-rich fresh fruit and vegetables. Heavy drinking raises blood pressure, so consume alcohol in moderation only (see Chapter 11).

Dealing with stress

If you have hypertension, there is very strong evidence that reducing stress, or coping better with it, can substantially reduce your blood pressure. You can do this only if you understand what stress is (see page 51) and how it contributes to hypertension, so that you can then avoid unnecessary stress.

The impact of stress that cannot be avoided altogether can still be reduced if you anticipate it and are prepared for it. If a stressful situation occurs suddenly, try to get it off your chest by talking it over with a friend, or work it off by going for a walk or having a game of tennis. Longer lasting stress can be reduced by learning to put a less threatening value on situations.

Most important of all, you can learn to relax. By learning breathing exercises, deep physical as well as mental relaxation, and by ensuring that you have adequate sleep, you can, to a large extent, help yourself. Exercise is also relaxing and refreshing, and increases your sense of well-being. All the above self-help measures are described in more detail in the self-help section, Chapters 10 to 14.

MEASURING YOUR BLOOD PRESSURE

If you have high blood pressure, you should make sure your blood pressure is checked regularly. In recent years, more and more people who have hypertension have been learning to take their own blood pressure. The technique can be learnt very quickly and, with a little practice, you can obtain very reliable readings more frequently and more conveniently at home than in a doctor's surgery. In addition to the convenience of monitoring your own blood pressure regularly, you can also gain a most important insight into its behaviour: what makes it go up; how long it takes to come down again; and how self-help measures, such as relaxation or weight loss, can reduce your blood pressure and by what degree.

Before buying an instrument to measure your own blood pressure, discuss with your doctor if he thinks it would be useful in your case. You will need to buy a stethoscope and a sphygmomanometer (see page 32) that is simple, accurate and reliable. The mercury sphygmomanometer is more reliable than the aneroid one in which the meter is like a dial of a small clock. Some instruments are now available with a built-in stethoscope and these are more convenient for home use. Since the endpiece of the stethoscope is secured inside the cuff, it leaves one hand free to pump the bulb without worrying about dislodging or displacing the stethoscope. Electronic sphygmomanometers have also now been developed which do not require you to have a stethoscope. The sounds of the artery oscillating are picked up by a small microphone that is built into the cuff and transformed into bleeps or flashing lights.

Sources of error

In surveys of hospital sphygmomanometers, it has been shown that as many as half are inaccurate, mainly because of poor maintenance. It is of vital importance, therefore, that your instrument is marketed by a reputable company (your doctor may be able to advise you) and that you make sure that it is regularly maintained.

The most common source of error, however, is you yourself. By taking your blood pressure at the wrong time, it is possible to obtain a falsely high measurement. The reading is likely to be higher than your usual blood pressure at rest if:

● You are anxious, nervous or upset about something
● You are in a hurry
● You are preoccupied with some other matter, however trivial
● You have just eaten a heavy meal, had a cigarette or a cup of coffee
● You have just performed some strenuous activity, such as climbing a flight of stairs.

CONCLUSION

To sum up, high blood pressure is very common and, if uncontrolled, can lead to several serious complications such as strokes, heart failure, angina, heart attacks and kidney failure. High blood pressure can be identified only by having it measured. Everyone should therefore have their blood pressure checked every five years, or more frequently if it is on the high side. Hypertension can be easily controlled, and complications thus averted. Your own contribution in this task is vital.

HOW TO TAKE YOUR BLOOD PRESSURE

Taking your blood pressure may look complicated but it is very easy to learn. Your doctor will advise you how often to take it. Generally it is a good idea to take it twice a day until you get used to the technique. After that, unless your blood pressure is very high, once a week will probably be sufficient. Try to take it at the same time of day each time. Sit down quietly for a while before taking it; don't hurry through the procedures, since this could make the reading inaccurate.

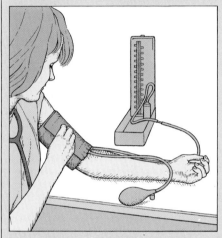

1 Place the sphygmomanometer on the table where you can see the scale clearly and put the stethoscope round your neck. Roll your sleeve right up and rest your arm on the table. (Use your left arm if you are right handed or your right arm if you are left handed.) Wrap the cuff round your arm just above the elbow; it should be firm but not tight.

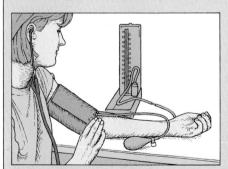

2 Put the ear pieces of the stethoscope in your ears. Feel for the brachial pulse with your fingers – the brachial artery runs down the inner side of your arm (see page 19).

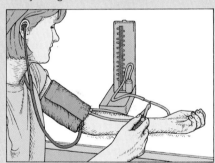

3 Position the end-piece of the stethoscope under the cuff against the brachial artery. If it is in the correct position, you will hear the pulse when you begin to inflate the cuff.

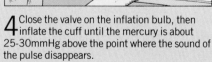

4 Close the valve on the inflation bulb, then inflate the cuff until the mercury is about 25-30mmHg above the point where the sound of the pulse disappears.

5 Open the valve slightly and release the pressure gradually until you can hear the pulse again. Note the measurement on the scale. This is the systolic pressure reading.

6 Continue deflating the cuff until the sound of the pulse disappears again. Note the measurement on the scale now; this is the diastolic pressure reading. Write down both readings and keep them for future reference.

8

Angina pectoris

Angina pectoris (from *angina* meaning strangling and *pectoris* meaning breast) is commonly known simply as angina and means pain in the chest. It is a tight, vice-like pain in the centre of the chest behind the breastbone, often radiating to one or both arms, or to the neck, throat and jaw. It occurs when the heart is not receiving enough oxygen to meet an increased demand. For example, when you run for a bus, have an argument with a colleague, or lose your temper with your spouse, your heart beats faster, your body becomes tense and your blood pressure rises. At times such as these, the heart is called upon to do extra work and the heart muscle temporarily needs more oxygen. A normal heart has no problem meeting this extra demand, but when one (or more) of the coronary arteries is narrowed, this may impede the flow of blood containing oxygen, so that there is insufficient oxygen to meet the demand and the heart "complains" by producing the pain known as angina.

A warning signal

This pain is your heart's distress signal – a built-in warning device which indicates that the heart has reached its maximum workload. Its onset means that you should stop and rest if you are over-exerting yourself, or calm down if you are feeling emotionally stressed. Except during these brief periods, the blood supply to the heart muscle is usually adequate. Angina does not in itself cause permanent damage to the heart muscle because the pain forces you to rest and the heart muscle once again receives enough oxygen and nourishment. The underlying coronary heart disease, however, continues to progress unless steps are taken to prevent it advancing further.

This chapter is intended to increase your understanding of angina, so that you can recognize when chest pain is angina and when it is not, and, most important of all, what steps you can take so that you can continue to enjoy your life to the fullest possible extent.

SIGNS AND SYMPTOMS

Angina is often described by patients simply as a "pain", but in fact it feels different to different people. If you have angina, your pain may feel like any one of the following descriptions, or a combination of several of these:

● Mild, vague discomfort in the centre of the chest, which may radiate to the left shoulder or arm

● Dull ache, pins and needles, heaviness or pains in the arms, usually more severe in the left arm

● Pain that feels like severe indigestion
● Heaviness, tightness, fullness, dull ache, intense pressure, a burning, vice-like, constricting, squeezing sensation in the chest, throat or upper abdomen
● Extreme tiredness, exhaustion or a feeling of collapse
● Shortness of breath
● A sense of foreboding or impending death accompanying chest discomfort
● Choking sensation
● Pains in the jaw, gums, teeth, throat or ear lobe
● Pains in the back or between the shoulder blades.

Angina can be so severe that you feel very frightened, or so mild that you tend to ignore it. It may occur in one of the places mentioned above or it may start at one place and spread to others. An attack does not last more than a minute or two – perhaps four to five minutes at most – though at the time it may feel much longer. As you rest, the pain slowly fades away, within a couple of minutes, or ten minutes at the most.

The Roman philosopher Seneca, who himself had angina, described it thus: "The attack is very short and like a storm. To have any other malady is only to be sick. To have this is to be dying." Angina patients have given the following descriptions of their experience:
● "It felt as if an elephant was sitting on my chest."

Angina pain
The pain generally starts at the centre of the chest and radiates out towards the left arm and some-times along the right arm and up the neck.

Site of pain

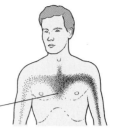

● "It was as if my chest was being held in a steel vice and someone was screwing it tighter and tighter."
● "I felt sick in my stomach, but it wasn't the usual feeling of sickness."
● "It felt like a cramp in my chest and at the same time there was a lump in my throat."
● "It was as if something inside my chest was going to explode. I was really frightened."
● "It was strange that I got toothache only when I walked uphill. I decided to see my dentist but he said that my teeth were perfect."
● "As I was climbing the stairs, I suddenly broke out in a cold sweat. My arms weighed a ton and I stopped dead still. Somehow it passed off within a few minutes."
● "I just felt a dull aching sensation in my chest."
● "At first I thought I had indigestion and I took some tablets, but then I realized that I was getting the pain even when I had had very little to eat."

DIFFERENT FORMS OF ANGINA

Brief anginal pain that comes on exertion and disappears fairly quickly on rest is known as stable angina. When angina also occurs during rest, it is known as unstable angina. The symptoms are usually severe and the coronary arteries are badly narrowed. The risk of developing a heart attack is somewhat higher

if you suffer from unstable angina. The pain may occur repeatedly, sometimes only once or twice a day, sometimes as many as ten to 20 times a day; occasionally it can wake you up, especially after a disturbing dream.

There is yet another type of angina, known as atypical or variant angina, in which pain occurs only when you are resting or asleep rather than during exertion. It is thought to occur as the result of coronary artery spasm, a sort of cramp that narrows the arteries.

It is not a heart attack

It is important for you to understand that angina and a heart attack are not the same thing. Angina is caused by a temporary shortage in the supply of blood, and therefore oxygen, to the heart in relation to the amount required, and the pain usually occurs during exercise or strong emotional stress. Stopping the exercise, or sitting down quietly, and sucking an angina tablet (see page 90) usually bring relief. But if the coronary arteries are so narrow that any part becomes completely blocked, thereby cutting off the blood supply to part of the heart for a prolonged period, that part of the heart muscle begins to die and a heart attack occurs. The pain is usually more severe than the pain of angina, lasts longer, and does not decrease on rest or on medication; other symptoms include sweating and nausea. (For more information on heart attacks, see Chapter 9).

Angina does not leave any permanent injury, whereas a heart attack does. Equally, having angina does not mean that a heart attack is inevitable, but you are twice as likely to have a heart attack in the future if you have angina. Unlike a heart attack, an episode of angina is not usually life-threatening.

WHAT CAUSES ANGINA?

The inside walls of coronary arteries are normally smooth and elastic, which allows them to constrict and expand and lets varying amounts of oxygenated blood, appropriate to the demand at the time, flow through them. As you get older, and particularly if the linings of the arteries are damaged as a result of cigarette smoking or high blood pressure, fatty deposits begin to cling to the walls. As these deposits, or plaques, build up, the internal diameter of the arteries becomes narrowed, restricting the flow of blood.

This process, known as atherosclerosis, is described in more detail in Chapter 6. Although atherosclerosis starts early in life, the process is so slow that it progresses for years before the arteries are narrowed enough to cause angina, which often occurs around middle age. Our reserve capacity is also such that two-thirds of the artery's diameter has to be blocked before angina can occur. As the heart is more frequently called upon to do extra work than any other organ or part of the body, it is not surprising that angina is a common consequence of atherosclerosis.

There is, needless to say, more to angina than atherosclerosis, and indeed, other heart conditions in which the heart muscle is starved of oxygen also cause angina. The reason that atherosclerosis tends to be given so much emphasis by doctors in this context is that it fits in with the mechanistic view of the body's workings and seems to offer theoretical hope of mechanical intervention. Unfortunately, however, human beings are more complex than this view suggests, and it is beginning to be realized that many other human factors have to be considered.

The nerve factor

First of all, the arteries are supplied with nerves, which allow them to be narrowed or widened on the direct command of the brain, especially the hypothalamus – an area at the centre of the brain that regulates the emotions. This control mechanism can be triggered off by the pressures of modern life, generating as they do aggression, hostility, never-ending deadlines, remorseless competition, unrest, insecurity and so on. If the arteries are narrowed through disease, the heart has to work harder than ever in times of stress and is in great need of blood containing oxygen. In addition, the chemicals that are released when you become emotional, such as adrenaline, noradrenaline and serotonin, can cause a further constriction of the coronary arteries. The pituitary gland, a small gland at the base of the brain, under the control of the hypothalamus, can signal the adrenal glands to increase their production of stress hormones such as corstisol and adrenaline still further.

Coronary spasm

Minute particles in the blood, called platelets, which play an essential role both in the clotting process and in repairing any damaged arterial walls, clump together more readily when the blood is full of the chemicals that are released during arousal. A raised level of these and other chemicals in the blood, including cortisol, is thought to be implicated in a condition known as coronary spasm, a contraction of one of

the coronary arteries that can lead to angina or even to a heart attack.

Coronary spasm encourages platelets to stick together and to the wall of the artery, while substances released by the platelets as they stick together further constrict the blood vessels. If there is already some narrowing of the arteries as a result of atherosclerosis, the nervous control mechanisms can drastically reduce the blood flow.

This vicious circle of events probably only scratches the surface of what is really going on. When people are very tense, they often overbreathe or hold their breath altogether, both of which can have a deleterious effect. Shallow, irregular but rapid breathing washes out carbon dioxide from the system and allows the blood to become over-oxygenated. Contrary to what one might expect, overloaded blood does not give up oxygen easily, and the amount of oxygen available to the heart is therefore reduced. Carbon dioxide is present in the blood as carbonic acid and when this is lost by overbreathing, the blood becomes alkaline, which leads to spasm of blood vessels, almost certainly in the brain but also in the heart.

Other causes

Although nervous and biochemical factors are more likely to affect those whose arteries are already narrowed by atherosclerosis, they also explain why some angina patients have normal

Spasm in a coronary artery
Sudden contraction of the muscle layer in the artery wall can cause blood platelets to stick together, temporarily restricting the flow of blood. The spasm may be relieved spontaneously and normal blood will return, or it may cause angina or a heart attack.

Normal blood flow

Spasm

Restricted blood flow

Blood cells including platelets

Spasm

Restricted blood flow beyond spasm

coronary arteries. It has been reported that up to 15 per cent of those who are referred for coronary artery bypass surgery (see page 93) have normal arteries. Conversely, many patients with severely constricted arteries have made brilliant recoveries from their angina and heart attacks, not only because they followed their doctor's advice about diet and drugs but also because they took their lives in their own hands and intuitively made the appropriate changes in lifestyle.

Unfortunately, many heart patients struggle relentlessly against the mounting pressures in their lives, and when confronted by the warning sign of angina, they tend to look upon it as a hostile agent and then ignore it completely. Rather than taking responsibility for preventing further attacks, they consider that it is a sign of weakness to accept defeat and prefer to carry on making a superhuman effort. Western culture is such that, while mechanical breakdown is accepted, making any emotional compromise is seen as a sign of weakness. Thus the warning signs of an essentially reversible condition are ignored and emotional resources overstretched, while the disease continues to progress.

What triggers off an attack?

As you become more familiar with angina, you will notice that certain activities are likely to bring on an attack. Some of the most common of these are:

● Physical exertion, such as walking uphill, rushing up the stairs, or running for a bus
● Smoking a cigarette or taking the dog for a walk after a heavy meal
● Walking in cold or hot and humid weather, especially if you are struggling against a strong wind
● Lifting and carrying heavy weights
● Shovelling snow
● Stress, fright, anxiety, anger, a heated argument or any other strong emotional tension or conflict
● Sexual intercourse, especially if it is with an extra-marital partner, when great passion, guilt or anxiety about your performance is involved
● Higher altitudes than those to which you are accustomed.

Not all chest pains are angina

Fortunately, not all chest pains are angina, or indeed any other serious condition. It is important, however, to distinguish between them as otherwise they can easily cause undue anxiety, which will certainly do no good, and may even increase your pain. Your symptoms may be due to:

● Tension or spasms in the chest wall muscles, which often produce a sharp, stabbing chest pain in a small area on one side of the chest; if the pain is on the left-hand side, it can be mistaken for heart disease
● Diseases of the stomach or other parts of the gastro-intestinal tract, ranging from indigestion, wind in the stomach or colitis to hiatus hernia, peptic ulcer and gall bladder disease
● Damage to the spine, caused by an old injury, a prolapsed disc or arthritis
● Inflammation or chill of the membranes surrounding the heart or lungs, known respectively as pericarditis and pleurisy
● Inflammation of one of the joints between a rib and the breastbone
● Anxiety, especially if a close member of the family or a colleague has died of a heart attack
● A defective valve in the heart, known as valve prolapse, which usually occurs in relatively young people
● Cardiac neurosis (see page 23).

DIAGNOSIS

Once you have experienced chest pain, you will want to know if it is angina. Your doctor will be helped tremendously by the history you provide. He will also give you a physical examination and carry out routine tests; and if necessary, he will arrange for special tests to confirm his suspicions.

History

This involves telling your doctor, as honestly and as accurately as possible, all the details about your symptoms, and answering a series of questions that he will ask you. You will need to tell him, for example, precisely where you felt the pain, what it was like, what you were doing before or while it occurred, and what you did to relieve it.

The doctor will also want to know if you had any other symptoms that may help him to distinguish angina from other conditions. It is essential that you neither minimize your symptoms, thinking they are unimportant, nor exaggerate them out of all proportion in the belief that otherwise the doctor won't take you seriously.

As well as your symptoms, the doctor will need to know about your general health over the years, your dietary and smoking habits, your relationships with your partner and other members of the family, the job you do, and how you are generally enjoying life. Do you feel that, most of the time at least, you have things under control, or do you find life an empty, joyless struggle, without any real hope? What is your emotional state? Do you feel irritable and anxious, or indifferent and depressed? Do you feel unusually exhausted? Have you been avoiding your responsibilities and keeping yourself to yourself, or are you dosing yourself with painkillers, alcohol, cigarettes and excessive coffee in order to cope with extra demands made on you? Your answers can help the doctor not only to make his diagnosis, but also to plan the most appropriate management of your condition.

Physical examination

This will almost certainly involve taking your pulse and blood pressure, listening to your heart and lungs with a stethoscope, and checking your weight. The doctor may also examine your abdomen and spine if that is pertinent to your history. His examination may tell him whether he should suspect any other conditions, but on its own it is not enough to diagnose angina or coronary heart disease. In other words, the history is more crucial than the examination, so it is essential that you give your doctor as much information as possible.

Routine tests

These tests are discussed more fully in Chapter 3. There are no blood or urine tests which will indicate whether or not your symptoms are due to angina, but they can tell if your blood level of fats is high (a risk factor) and, if your blood pressure is high, they can tell if this is due to kidney disease or if it has caused kidney damage. You may have a chest X-ray, which gives a good idea of the size and structure of your heart.

You will almost certainly have an electrocardiogram (ECG), see page 37. This picks up electrical signals of your heart's activity, which may reveal any disturbance in the blood supply to the heart or significant irregularities in the heart beats. It can confirm a diagnosis of angina or coronary heart disease, but about 60 per cent of patients who have angina have a perfectly normal ECG.

Exercise stress test

This test, sometimes called an exercise ECG or heart stress test, shows how your heart reacts to a specific amount of exercise. It is usually done to confirm or reject a tentative diagnosis of angina based on medical history, examination and routine tests. It can also tell the doctor how much exercise you can do without getting angina and without changes in the ECG. Sometimes, however, you may have angina pain without any changes in the ECG pattern.

The stress test is increasingly becoming a routine part of regular private check-ups. Most doctors recommend the stress test before taking up jogging, marathons or any other strenuous exercise. It is also a part of the rehabilitation programme after a heart attack.

The test is carried out in appropriately equipped consulting rooms of heart specialists or in a nearby hospital laboratory. You will be told whether to take your routine medication before the test, and for how long before the test not to eat. Wear loose, comfortable clothes and good walking or jogging shoes.

How the test is carried out

You will be connected to an ECG machine and a blood pressure cuff will be applied to your arm. Your blood pressure will be measured before the test and at intervals throughout. Some laboratories also measure the amount of oxygen used during the test.

The exercise is done on a treadmill or on a stationary bicycle. A treadmill is a power-driven belt that rotates around a small platform. The incline of the platform and the rate at which the belt moves can be increased as necessary. You will be asked to walk on the belt while holding on to a rail, at first slowly and on the level, then gradually faster and faster, and more and more uphill. When a stationary bicycle is used, the amount of effort you are required to make is increased either by pedalling faster, or by having to push the pedals harder to maintain the same speed.

You will be watched carefully while you do the stress test. Your ECG will be constantly visible on an oscilloscope, which looks like a television screen, and your blood pressure will be measured every minute. The test is usually continued until you reach a "target" heart rate which is based on your age and general condition.

The doctor may stop the test if he sees certain changes in your electrocardiogram, if your blood pressure either rises too high or fails to rise adequately, or if you become short of breath. You may stop the test yourself if you feel unduly tired, have chest discomfort, or feel short of breath. The test is quite safe when carried out by properly qualified people. Always remember, the doctor is there to help you. You may feel tired after taking the test, just as you would after any exercise.

SPECIAL TESTS FOR ANGINA

With your history, examination and the routine tests described above, there should be no difficulty in diagnosing angina. In some patients, however, it is necessary to know more about the underlying coronary heart disease and one or more of the following tests may be proposed. They are done for a variety of reasons, all of which are closely linked to coronary heart disease and its complications. Angina is just one of those complications, others include rhythm

BICYCLE STRESS TEST

This test monitors the activity of your heart while you are performing fairly strenuous exercise. Since it is always carried out under medical supervision, there is no danger to your health. You can stop the test if any of your symptoms recur.

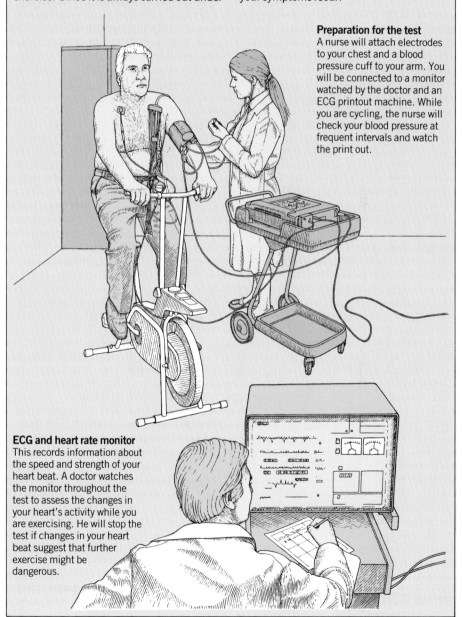

Preparation for the test
A nurse will attach electrodes to your chest and a blood pressure cuff to your arm. You will be connected to a monitor watched by the doctor and an ECG printout machine. While you are cycling, the nurse will check your blood pressure at frequent intervals and watch the print out.

ECG and heart rate monitor
This records information about the speed and strength of your heart beat. A doctor watches the monitor throughout the test to assess the changes in your heart's activity while you are exercising. He will stop the test if changes in your heart beat suggest that further exercise might be dangerous.

disturbance and previously undetected heart attack.

Ambulatory monitoring of ECG

As the name implies, this is a continuous ECG recording for as long as 24 hours while you continue with your usual activities. It is sometimes called "Holter" monitoring after the man who originated the method.

Four small metal discs, known as electrodes, are taped to your chest and wires from these are connected to a small battery-operated tape recorder which you wear attached either to a belt or a shoulder strap. It takes about an hour to attach the electrodes, to connect the recorder and to check that your heart activity is being recorded.

You then go about your usual daily activities – except for swimming or bathing, which could dislodge the electrodes. You are asked to keep a diary of your activities, noting down the time of days you are engaged in each one. You should also record any symptoms you

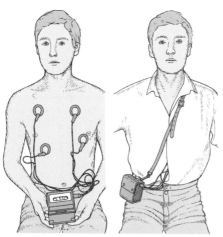

Wearing a 24-hour heart monitor
Four electrodes are taped to your chest, then connected to a tape recorder, left. You carry the monitor in a pouch attached to your belt and/or a shoulder strap, right.

experience, again noting down the exact time you have them. At the end of the recording period, you return to the laboratory where the electrodes will be removed and your diary collected.

The ECG tape is then analyzed by a special machine. Selected parts of the record are printed and matched against the activities and symptoms you have recorded in your diary.

Ambulatory monitoring is especially useful to detect rhythm disturbance (slow, fast or irregular heartbeats) which only occurs intermittently. The correct diagnosis of the exact type of rhythm disturbance is very important because dangerous rhythm disturbance, requiring prompt treatment, may be present without any specific symptoms, while a harmless type of rhythm disturbance may cause annoying symptoms. For example, dizzy spells and fainting attacks, for which there is no apparent cause, can both be due to rhythm disturbances, and ambulatory monitoring is useful in detecting them.

This test is also useful in studying the effect of medicines and in evaluating the functioning of implanted cardiac pacemakers (see page 116).

Echo-cardiography

Most of us are familiar with the echo when we shout in a large empty room. Echo-cardiography makes use of this property of sound waves. It uses waves of such high frequency, however, that they cannot be heard and are known as "ultrasound". When these sound waves are directed to the heart, the pattern of the returning echo outlines the size and motion of various parts of the heart muscle. These echoes are translated by the ultrasound machine into a picture on a television screen and sometimes also on to a tape or video-cassette that can be played back later.

The test is simple, takes about half an hour and requires no preparation except undressing to the waist. The technician spreads a jelly-like cream on your chest and then holds a small device called a transducer in various places over your heart. The transducer sends out ultra-sound signals and receives echoes back from the heart which it sends to the recording machine.

The muscular walls of the heart chambers normally contract in perfect harmony but if there is a poor blood supply or scar tissue from a previous heart attack, some areas of wall that are relatively immobile (known as areas of akinesia) will be detected. This test is also useful in detecting a valve defect, as well as diagnosing many other heart conditions. It is a simple and completely safe procedure, which can be repeated frequently in order to follow the progression of a particular disease.

Heart scanning

There are several different types of scan, including thalium, technitium and muga scans, in which a radioactive chemical called a radio-isotope is injected into a vein. The substance then travels through the bloodstream into the heart. The rays that are emitted by the radioactive substance are pictured by a special camera or monitor. These tests will indicate which areas of the heart muscle are short of blood when you exercise. They are particularly useful in the diagnosis of both angina and heart attack; in assessing the suitability of patients for coronary artery bypass surgery; and in monitoring progress after treatment.

These scans are perfectly harmless, and radioactivity disappears quickly from the body. The only discomfort you will feel is the prick of the injection. Since this test involves some exposure to radioactivity, however, you should not have a scan if you are pregnant.

Cardiac catheterization and coronary angiography

A coronary angiograph is a type of X-ray which shows where a coronary artery is narrowed or blocked and reveals more about the general condition of the heart muscle and how well the heart is functioning. It is particularly valuable when coronary artery bypass surgery is considered. In the large majority of angina patients whose diagnosis is not in doubt, and whose condition is satisfactorily controlled by medical therapy, this invasive and uncomfortable procedure is not usually performed.

A long, narrow, flexible plastic tube (catheter) is inserted into an accessible vein or artery in the leg or arm and guided into the heart. The pressure is measured in each chamber of the heart, and blood samples are taken for testing.

The catheter is then guided to a point near the origin of the coronary arteries,

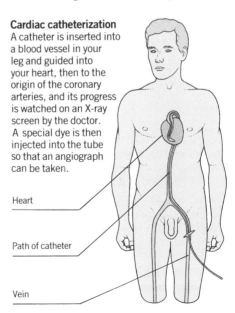

Cardiac catheterization
A catheter is inserted into a blood vessel in your leg and guided into your heart, then to the origin of the coronary arteries, and its progress is watched on an X-ray screen by the doctor. A special dye is then injected into the tube so that an angiograph can be taken.

Heart

Path of catheter

Vein

a special dye that shows up on X-rays is injected into each coronary artery, and a series of X-rays, or angiographs, is taken. Dye may also be injected into the various chambers of the heart while a film is made to study the size and function of the heart chambers. Abnormal communication between chambers or leaky heart valves may also be seen.

This procedure takes about an hour and you will be sedated, but conscious throughout. You will be kept in hospital overnight. You will feel a burning sensation throughout your body and have a bitter taste in your mouth for a few seconds when the dye is injected. You may have a headache or nausea for a short time. There is also a risk, albeit very small, of the procedure triggering off a heart attack. Depending on the results of the investigation, you will be told whether or not surgery is needed.

WHAT TO DO IF YOU HAVE ANGINA

If you have angina, you must get to know your condition. Find out what kind of activities or situations bring on attacks, and what the attacks feel like. Ask yourself whether it is possible to avoid these situations. Remember how long your attacks usually last and how soon after rest the pain or discomfort fades away. Does medication prevent angina attacks? Can you stop attacks by avoiding heavy meals, by spacing out your physical activities, avoiding anything very strenuous, or by learning to control your emotions?

Danger signs

As you become familiar with the pattern of your angina, you should be able to recognize any changes in this pattern.

The signs, listed right, do not necessarily signify a heart attack, but if you are uncertain, you should consult your doctor without delay. If the discomfort is particularly severe or unusual, and you cannot contact your doctor immediately, get someone to drive you to the nearest casualty department or call 999 for an ambulance. Only qualified people can tell if there is cause for concern. Don't worry if it turns out to be a false alarm. It is better to be safe than sorry. Make sure that you always have your doctor's telephone number or the hospital telephone number handy.

What to do during an attack

Stop whatever you are doing and stand still or, preferably, sit down. Take slow, deep breaths to increase your intake of oxygen. Your heart will soon slow down and the discomfort will pass off. If you have trinitrates (see opposite), suck one of these immediately.

Angina attacks do not usually last more than five minutes. If an attack lasts for more than ten minutes, call for a doctor or an ambulance.

IMPORTANT

Get immediate attention if your pain:
- Occurs more frequently than usual
- Is brought on by less exertion than usual
- Lasts longer than usual
- Is not helped by resting or your usual medication
- Occurs in unusual circumstances
- Seems more severe or widespread
- Feels different in other ways
- Persists after you have been discharged from hospital after a heart attack
- Begins to develop at night and to wake you up from a deep sleep
- Persists for more than 10 to 20 minutes
- Is severe enough to cause cold sweats.

DRUG TREATMENT

If you have angina, you will probably be prescribed at least one drug. Each drug is likely to have a different function. Some drugs improve the flow of blood through the coronary arteries, while others reduce the strain on the heart.

Whenever you are prescribed a drug, you should know:
● Its name, bearing in mind that some drugs go under more than one name
● How it affects your condition
● When and how often you must take it
● How much you should take each time
● Whether you are allowed by your doctor to increase or decrease the prescribed dose
● The possible side-effects
● Whether you should avoid taking other non-prescribed medication or alcohol while on this drug
● If it is likely to interfere with driving or other activities
● That most heart drugs are not addictive, but if you are at all worried you should ask your doctor
● That several drugs, while doing you good, do not necessarily make you feel better immediately.

Take your medication regularly

If you have been prescribed drugs, you must always take them regularly and if you have any queries or side-effects, discuss them with your doctor. Even if you feel perfectly well, do not stop taking your medication without consulting your doctor; stopping certain medication abruptly can cause problems.

Commonly prescribed drugs for angina are nitrates, beta-blockers and calcium antagonists. Remember that the drugs prescribed for angina are only for the relief of pain: they do nothing to the underlying disorder, which must be tackled by changes in lifestyle. Relief

from pain provided by the drug could make you lose sight of this essential task.

NITRATES

A small amount of nitroglycerine, which is the basis of dynamite, can relax the smooth fibres of the blood vessels, thus allowing coronary arteries as well as other arteries in the body to dilate. These effects lessen the arteries' resistance to blood flow, enabling the blood to move more easily and in a greater quantity, thus relieving an acute attack of angina pain. Since other arteries in the body will also dilate, the drug has an unfortunate tendency to produce flushing and headaches. You will, however, be glad to know that, once you have taken nitrates for a few days, the headaches are likely to become less severe and may even disappear altogether.

Glyceryl trinitrate

This is a short-acting drug prescribed in the form of a small tablet which is kept under the tongue for absorption: the blood supply under the tongue is very rich so the drug is absorbed quickly, giving relief within a minute or two. If you have an angina attack, stand still or sit down and suck one of your tablets; if the chest pain is not relieved after two or three minutes, suck another one. Always carry a fresh supply of tablets and keep them in an amber-coloured bottle, which prevents them from deteriorating in sunlight. Do not mix them with other tablets or keep them out in a pill box. Do not take them after a heavy meal or with an alcoholic drink, as they might make you feel faint.

Trinitrate has recently been made available in the form of an ointment or "transdermal" sticky patch, which is applied to the skin anywhere on the body; the drug is absorbed through the skin over 24 hours.

Dinitrates and mononitrates

These drugs are prescribed for the prevention of angina attacks rather than for the relief of an acute episode. They are slower to act, have a more prolonged effect, and are taken three to four times a day. Dinitrates and mononitrates are more common than trinitrates or tetranitrates, although the emergency drug you carry with you is a trinitrate.

BETA-BLOCKERS

These are used to prevent angina, or at least to reduce the severity of an attack.

They reduce the work of the heart by regulating the heart beat and slowing it down, as well as by reducing blood pressure; the amount of oxygen which is required by the heart is thereby reduced. They are described more fully in Chapter 7, under the treatment of high blood pressure (see page 74). They must be taken exactly as prescribed, as there could be alarming results (even the precipitation of a heart attack) if you stop taking them abruptly.

CALCIUM ANTAGONISTS

These drugs can help prevent angina in two ways: they relax and dilate the coronary arteries, thus allowing more

DRUGS USED FOR ANGINA

NITRATES

Generic name	Trade example	Slow-release preparations	Other forms
isosorbide dinitrate	Cedocard	Cedocard retard	Sobichew (to be chewed)
	Isordil	Isoket retard	Isordil (to be taken under the tongue)
	Sorbitrate	Soni-slow	—
	Vascardin	—	—
isosorbide moninitrate	Elantan, ISMO, Monit, Monocedocard	—	—
glyceryl trinitrate	Trinitrin	Sustac	Suscard buccal
	—	Nitrocontin continus	Nitrolingual spray
	—	—	Percutol ointment
	—	—	Transiderm nitro patch (rubbed on the skin)
tetranitrate	Mycardol	—	—
pentaerythritol	Peritrite	—	—

CALCIUM ANTAGONISTS		RELATIVELY NEW DRUGS	
Generic name	Trade example	Generic name	Trade example
nifedipine	Azdalat	lidoflazine	Clinium
verapamil	Cordilox, Securon, Berkatens	captopril	Capoten
diltiazem	Tildiem	enalapril	Innovace

blood and oxygen to reach the heart muscle, and they help the heart muscle to use the oxygen and nutrients carried in the blood more efficiently. In larger doses they also reduce blood pressure (see page 76). They are particularly helpful if angina is thought to be linked to coronary artery spasm (see page 83). They tend to cause fluid retention and may thus give rise to swollen ankles.

OTHER MEDICATIONS

New drugs are constantly being developed. Pexid, for example, is useful if other drugs fail in severe angina; it does, however, produce more side-effects than others, such as pins and needles or numbness in the limbs, muscle weakness and liver damage; it may also precipitate diabetes, and eye examinations are necessary to ensure that there is no damage to the retina.

You may be given drugs to control high blood pressure, or to regulate heart rhythm if there are heart irregularities, or drugs to strengthen the heart beats if your heart has weakened (heart failure).

DRUGS IN PERSPECTIVE

If you continue to live in the way you lived before angina started, no drugs are going to cure you. What you can do for yourself, on the other hand, is far more impressive, as the following story, cited in a recent medical journal, illustrates. A group of angina patients retreated into a rural setting for 24 days, during which they lived on a vegetarian diet and exercised and meditated for five hours daily; the number of angina attacks fell from an average of 10 per day to one; the amount of exercise they could do before getting angina was increased, on average, by 44 per cent; their level of blood cholesterol fell by approximately 20 per cent, and many patients were able to reduce, and some to stop, their medication for angina or high blood pressure.

The moral of this story is that anti-anginal drugs should be seen as agents that help you over a particular hurdle which brings on disabling pain; they are only a temporary stop-gap. The most important lesson to learn is not to withdraw from the world but to look more objectively at the way you have been treating yourself. Learn to relax and to reduce your arousal level, to treat your body with respect and to improve your general health and stamina (see pages 150 to 180). Too great a reliance on drugs may hinder your efforts to live within the limits of your pain and to preserve your physical, psychological and emotional fitness for your life.

SURGERY

When the pain of angina attacks cannot be controlled by the different means described so far, surgery is considered. There are two types of operation available: coronary artery bypass is the more common; angioplasty is a relatively new technique but is a minor operation. If it is unsuccessful, you can still have a bypass operation.

While surgery will provide relief from intractable angina, it is not a cure for the disease and you will still need to control the underlying disease through changes in your lifestyle. Surgical intervention is a treatment of last resort.

CORONARY ARTERY BYPASS

In this operation, a vein from another part of the body – usually the leg – is used to construct a detour around a diseased coronary artery. Thus the operation does not cure the underlying cause of the coronary artery disease, but it relieves the pain of angina by restoring the blood flow to the heart muscles which have been deprived of it.

What are the risks?

With experienced surgical teams, the death rate is below 3 per cent. The risk is greater if the disease is widespread and if the heart muscle is already weakened. A heart attack may occasionally occur after the operation, if the grafted artery becomes blocked. No two people are the same and, if you are going to have a bypass operation, you should not hesitate to discuss all the pros and cons with your doctor and your specialist.

How many bypasses?

Coronary artery disease can affect one, two or all three coronary arteries (see page 17). Several grafts may therefore be carried out during the operation.

About 20 per cent of patients who are considered for surgery have only one diseased vessel, in which case, unless it is the left main coronary artery, bypass surgery is not really indicated. In 50 per cent of patients who are considered for the operation, there are two diseased vessels. And in 30 per cent, the disease affects all three arteries (triple vessel disease). Triple vessel disease and disease of the left main coronary artery before it splits into two branches are the most serious conditions.

What the operation entails

An incision is made down the length of the breastbone to expose the heart. You are connected to a heart-lung machine, which takes over the function of your heart and lungs during the operation.

A small incision will be made in your leg, and a length of vein removed. One end of this length of vein is sewn on to the aorta, the main blood vessel leading from the heart, near the origin of your coronary arteries, and the other end is sewn into the coronary artery beyond the narrowed or blocked segment. The grafted vein then becomes the new artery through which the blood can flow freely beyond the obstruction. The latter is thus bypassed. The whole procedure usually takes about four to five hours – it may take longer if several bypasses are being carried out.

Recovery from the operation

After the operation you will spend a few days, on average between two and five, in the intensive-care unit (ICU), during which time your heart will be carefully monitored and you will be given fluid, in the form of glucose or salt water, and blood through intravenous drips. You will probably feel very sore in your chest, neck and back, and may even be confused about where you are. Pain-relieving drugs are given as necessary.

You may need to be given oxygen through a tube leading into your windpipe. You may also need the help of a respirator for a day or two, which moves air in and out of your lungs through the oxygen tube in your windpipe. It ensures that you are breathing deeply and expanding your lungs, and is removed as soon as you can breathe unaided.

Tubes are placed around your heart to drain air and fluid, and are connected to a vacuum container at the side of the bed; they are removed after a couple of days. For a day or so you will have a catheter in your bladder so that urine and kidney function can be measured.

Your immediate family will be allowed to visit you, but you will not be able to speak because of the breathing tubes. However, nurses are very skilled at non-verbal communication.

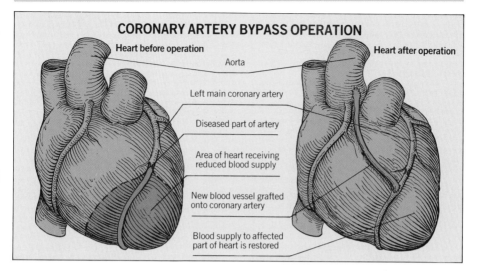

CORONARY ARTERY BYPASS OPERATION

Heart before operation

Heart after operation

Aorta

Left main coronary artery

Diseased part of artery

Area of heart receiving reduced blood supply

New blood vessel grafted onto coronary artery

Blood supply to affected part of heart is restored

While you are in the ICU you will have daily chest X-rays and ECGs, and your blood pressure and pulse will be taken several times a day. You will be asked to do foot and leg exercises as soon as possible after surgery. On the day after the operation, you may be allowed to sit on the edge of the bed. By the second day you may sit in a chair, and you may even take a few steps.

A physiotherapist will encourage you to take deep breaths and even to cough frequently so as to reduce the chances of post-operative pneumonia. All these exercises and activities are essential to hasten your recovery, although you may feel that you would prefer to rest.

Post-operative progress

If your condition is stable, you have no complications and can begin to care for yourself, you will be transferred to a general surgical ward after two to five days. By the time you are transferred, all the tubes will be out, you will be eating, and more activities will gradually be encouraged. How long you stay in hospital will depend on many factors, but it is usually around ten to 14 days.

Convalescence

Most patients need to convalesce at home for between three and six weeks. The immediate recovery period may be both physically and emotionally trying and it may be several months before you make a full recovery. However, you may notice marked improvements in symptoms within a few days.

The physical constraints and problems of psychological and social readjustment you will probably face are similar to those experienced after a heart attack. These are discussed more fully in the next chapter.

How effective is the operation?

Most people with severe angina will have their pain completely or partially controlled, at least at first. However, since a bypass does not cure the disease, the initial benefit begins to diminish after a while, which may be months or years. Thus the self-help measures recommended below, and in Chapters 10 to 14 are very important if the benefit is to last. Bypass surgery probably does not prolong life, and the operation is therefore of no value if your angina is

95

well controlled on drugs, but it could be invaluable if your angina cannot be controlled by medical therapy.

ANGIOPLASTY

This procedure, known in full as trans-luminal balloon coronary angioplasty, is occasionally used in some hospitals. It entails "squashing" the atherosclerotic plaques with balloons. A very thin balloon catheter is inserted into an artery in the arm or leg under general anaesthetic. The catheter is guided, under X-ray, just beyond the narrowed coronary artery. The balloon is then inflated with fluid for a few seconds and the fatty plaques are squashed against the artery wall. The balloon is then deflated and drawn out.

This technique is much simpler, cheaper and faster than coronary artery bypass surgery, entailing only a few days in hospital. Exactly how long it takes depends on where – and in how many places – the artery is narrowed. It is most suitable when the disease is limited to the left anterior descending branch of the coronary artery, but some plaques are so hard that it is simply not possible to squash them successfully.

SELF-HELP

The aim is to strike a balance between the demand put on the heart and the supply of blood available through the narrowed coronary arteries, and to halt the progress of the underlying disease. See Chapters 10 to 14 for more details.

Work

Limit your exertions to the point beyond which you know, through your experience, angina pain is likely to occur. Some angina patients can do as much work as they did before developing angina, as long as they do it just a bit more slowly and have brief periods of rest from time to time. Try to delegate more, reassess your priorities and learn to pace yourself. If you have no control over the rate of work you do, you may have to change your job.

Exercise

It may sound contradictory that, on the one hand, you are told to limit your exertion and, on the other, you are told to take regular exercise, but the more exercise you take – within your limits – the better it is for you. It will help your heart and body to get fitter (see pages 170 to 171), so that gradually you will be able to do more and more before the onset of an attack of angina.

Exercise can be divided into two categories: isotonic and isometric. You should limit yourself to isotonic exercises, in which one group of muscles is contracted while the opposite group is relaxed. Gentle examples of this type of exercise include walking, swimming at a leisurely pace and yoga; more strenuous examples are cycling and jogging.

As a general rule, however, remember that if you are not accustomed to regular exercise or have not done any for a few days, it is essential that you start gently and increase the amount very gradually, even if you do not experience chest pain. If you experience any chest pain, you must stop immediately and stand still, or sit down, until it passes. Exercise is discussed in greater detail in Chapter 14.

Weight loss

Every extra kilo you carry means additional and unnecessary strain on your heart. Losing weight not only reduces that strain, but is also likely to lower blood pressure – thus reducing the strain on your heart still further. There is no easy way to lose weight other than to eat less than your normal intake and to cut down on fatty and sugary foods which are nutritionally low, yet expensive in terms of calories. This is discussed in more detail in Chapter 10.

Diet
Even if you don't need to lose weight, it is wise, if you have angina, to eat fewer animal fats and foods high in cholesterol, such as fatty meat, lard, suet, butter, cream and hard cheese, as well as eggs, prawns and offal. Cholesterol and other fats have been implicated in the process of atherosclerosis and they should be eaten sparingly. Cut down on the amount of salt you eat (see page 131). Aim to eat more fibre, by increasing your intake of wholegrain cereal products, pulses, wholemeal bread and fresh fruits and vegetables.

Alcohol, tea and coffee
Alcohol in moderation does no harm and you may continue to have one or two standard drinks a day (see page 138) if you are used to doing so. Alcohol does contain calories, however, and you should remember this if you are trying to lose weight. You can drink as much mineral water, fruit juice and ordinary or herb tea as you like, but no more than two cups of coffee a day.

Cigarettes·
Smoking stimulates the heart to beat faster, constricts blood vessels and generally increases the work that your heart has to do. If you have been told you have angina, resolve to give up smoking (see Chapter 12). This will not be easy, but it is well worth the effort.

Stress
You should avoid those heated arguments and emotional situations that you know will make your blood pressure rise and may even bring on an attack of angina. If is is not possible to avoid them altogether, try to anticipate them and prevent an attack by sucking an angina tablet a few minutes beforehand. A certain amount of stress is necessary to give your life zest, but a constant battle with pressures of work, anxiety and aggression can be harmful and, in the long run, your heart may suffer.

Relaxation
There are several simple ways of helping your mind and body to relax which will be discussed in greater detail on pages 154 to 169. Briefly, however, the next time you feel tense, sit or lie down quietly, close your eyes and breathe slowly and deeply through your nose, making each exhalation long, soft and steady. Always have adequate sleep.

Sexual activity
Sexual intercourse may bring on an angina attack, but the chronic frustration of abstinence may produce more tension than the brief strain of intercourse. If you do find that intercourse precipitates angina, either suck an angina tablet beforehand or let your partner take the more active role.

CONCLUSION
Providing that you take care of yourself and follow your doctor's advice, there is every reason to be optimistic. Even if your activities are slightly restricted, you are certainly not an invalid.

Once you understand your angina, and have learned to control attacks with drugs and the self-help measures already discussed, you should have many years of active and enjoyable life.

9
Heart attack

The heart is the most important organ in the body; without it the rest of the body would not receive any oxygen or nutrition (see page 12). A heart attack is a condition in which damage occurs to part of the heart muscle (myocardium) as a result of a sudden extreme shortage of blood. This is a medical emergency because when a heart attack occurs there may be an interruption in the flow of blood around the body. A number of other terms are used to describe it, for instance coronary thrombosis, coronary occlusion, or simply coronary. Doctors usually call it myocardial infarction, or MI for short.

A sudden reduction in blood supply to the heart can occur when one of the coronary arteries becomes temporarily blocked, either by a spasm – a tightening of the coronary artery – or by a blood clot – thrombus –(see also pages 64 and 83). That part of the heart muscle which is normally supplied by the blocked artery ceases to function properly. As soon as a spasm is spontaneously relieved, the symptoms clear up completely and the heart muscle begins to function quite normally again. This is often called crescendo angina, or coronary insufficiency.

If, on the other hand, the blood supply to the heart is completely cut off, the cells undergo a permanent change within only a couple of hours and that part of the heart muscle degenerates or is permanently destroyed. This dead muscle is called an infarct.

WHAT ARE THE SYMPTOMS?

These vary from one person to another. A heart attack may begin as a dull ache, a vague discomfort or a feeling of heaviness in the centre of the chest. Sometimes a heart attack causes such minimal discomfort that it is mistaken for indigestion, or it may even pass unnoticed. In this case the only way it will be detected is when you have an ECG for some other, quite unrelated reason.

It may, on the other hand, be the worst pain you have ever experienced – a feeling of severe constriction, or a squeezing, vice-like pain in the chest, throat or abdomen. You may come out in hot or cold sweats, feel very weak in the legs and may be so frightened that you experience a sense of impending doom. You may feel more comfortable sitting than lying down, and you may be so breathless that you cannot relax. You may feel dizzy and nauseous or you may actually vomit. You may even collapse and pass out. Any of the symptoms of angina (see pages 80 to 81) can be present, but they tend to last longer.

When does it occur?
A heart attack can strike at any time of day or night. It may happen suddenly, or it may have been preceded by hours, or even days, of feeling under the weather. You may have experienced increasingly frequent and prolonged episodes of angina, or this may be the first indication that there is anything wrong with your heart. It is quite likely that you have been under a great deal of pressure, either at work or at home.

EARLY WARNING SIGNS

It is a misconception, however, that a heart attack strikes as a bolt from the blue. It is the catastrophic culmination of a long process of decline, frequently involving emotional upheavals, physiological turmoil and mental exhaustion. There are ample warnings if you are perceptive but it is, of course, possible that you have completely overlooked – or tried to ignore – the signs.

The warning signs are so subjective and so subtle that even your doctor, who is trained to measure things objectively, may miss them. If you have one or more of the obvious risk factors, such as high blood pressure or a high level of blood cholesterol, or if you smoke, your doctor may have advised you to stop smoking or to change your diet, and have prescribed pills to lower your blood pressure. But it is equally likely that you do not have any of these risk factors, in which case your vague feelings of ill-health may have been dismissed as insignificant.

Why are they so difficult to see?
One of the reasons for this is the difficulty in measuring people's feelings. When psychologists have tried to unravel these feelings through the use of questionnaires, some surprising facts have come to light. One such questionnaire, for example, was filled in by 3,570 male civil servants in Rotterdam, and revealed that 562 of them felt exhausted and depressed. Over the next three months, six of them had heart attacks. Five of these were from the group of exhausted and depressed men, who thus had a 27 times greater risk of having a heart attack. Admittedly the numbers are small, but the difference is nevertheless striking. Before a heart attack strikes, victims often feel that they have reached a dead end, that the future is bleak, and that physical and emotional strains are too great to handle.

Everyone feels depressed at times. The difference in those who have a heart attack is probably best explained by the human function curve put forward by cardiologist Dr Peter Nixon, of the Charing Cross Hospital, London.

At first our performance is increased in direct proportion to the mental effort (arousal) we expend in coping with everyday life. Once a peak is reached, however, there comes a point of diminishing returns. Just before the

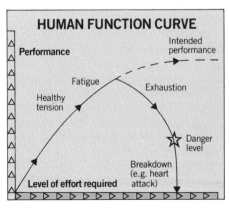

HUMAN FUNCTION CURVE

peak is reached, fatigue sets in and a relatively big increase in arousal is required to increase performance. Further efforts worsen the performance and cause exhaustion and depression.

If an individual does not spot the danger signal, distress or a breakdown will occur. A heart attack is one such breakdown. There are some who enjoy living dangerously at the top of the curve but have a deep sense of self-protection and know exactly when to

pull back. But there are others who live constantly beyond their healthy means in a state of chronic ill-health and may stay there for years until a sudden crisis pushes them into deeper trouble. And there are still others who have always lived a modest life, remaining on the upwards slope for most of their lives, when a catastrophe or a series of un-accustomed blows over a short period pulls them over the hump and plunges them into a breakdown.

DIAGNOSIS

A doctor will have a reasonably good idea from your symptoms whether or not they are indicative of a heart attack. His suspicions may be strengthened by your appearance, the level of your blood pressure, and the sound of your heart.

The doctor may also arrange for an ECG and blood test, but if you are still in pain he will probably give you a painkilling injection before he examines you. This is because frightening pain can send you into deeper shock, which may cause heart failure. It can also have long-term psychological effects. The first ECG may not show any signs of heart attack and the test may need to be repeated. Occasionally it still fails to show any change, in which case diagnosis will rely on a blood test.

The heart, like all other body cells, contains special chemicals known as enzymes. When damage occurs to the heart cells, enzymes are released into the bloodstream. The level of some of the enzymes is raised immediately after a heart attack, but the enzymes then break down early and are therefore no longer discernible after a day or two; other enzymes are released several hours or days later and remain in the blood for days or even weeks.

How serious is it?
This depends on the actual area of heart muscle that was destroyed, your age, any previous history of heart attack, the general condition of your heart, the presence or absence of any serious complications, and your overall physical and mental health. If the size of the infarct is fairly small, the heart's pumping ability is not seriously affected and the heart continues to beat regularly, there is every chance that you will make a full recovery and return to normal health.

If the size of the damaged area is large and the heart is having difficulty in pumping blood through the body, the condition must be brought swiftly under control by prompt treatment with oxygen and drugs. During a heart attack the rhythm of the heart may become disturbed, and this is exacerbated by certain chemicals, such as adrenaline and noradrenaline, which are released as a result of fear and panic. This rhythm disturbance may be transient and pass off without any further trouble. It may, on the other hand, herald a much more dangerous rhythm disturbance, which, unless treated, can lead to loss of consciousness and can even cause the heart to stop beating altogether.

FIRST AID FOR A HEART ATTACK

Correct treatment of a person who is having a heart attack can save his life. Even if you think the heart has stopped, start pumping it artificially by giving chest compression; you may be able to keep the blood supply going until the ambulance arrives. Here is an outline of the treatment you should give. These techniques can and should be learnt from the British Red Cross Society, St John's Ambulance, St Andrew's Ambulance Association in Scotland, or The Royal Life Saving Society (see page 187 for details).

WHAT TO DO

If you see someone collapse, establish first of all whether he is conscious or unconscious. Shake him gently by the shoulders and ask him a question. Give him a simple command such as "squeeze my hand" or "open your eyes". Give him a few seconds to respond.

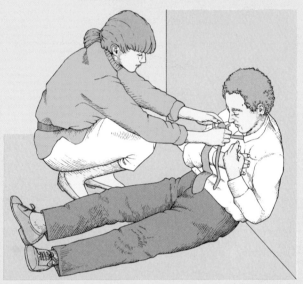

If he is conscious

Gently help him into a semi-sitting position with his head and shoulders raised and his knees bent. This is the best position for the heart to work.
■ Loosen clothing around the neck, chest and waist.
■ Make sure he is warm. If he is cold, cover him with blankets but do not give him a hot-water bottle or electric blanket because it will draw blood away from the heart and other vital organs to the surface.
■ Do not give him anything by mouth, including brandy or aspirin.

■ Do not move him unless it is absolutely essential for reasons of safety.
■ Stay with him to reassure and calm him until the doctor or ambulance arrives.

If he is unconscious

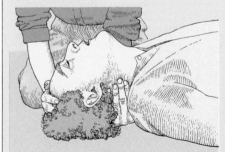

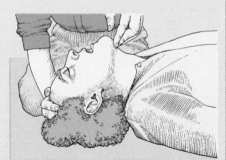

1 Lay him flat on the ground and tilt his head back as far as possible by placing one hand on his forehead and one under his neck.

2 Then, still supporting his forehead with one hand, push his chin up and forward with the other. This will open all the air passages. Now check breathing, see overleaf.

CHECKING BREATHING

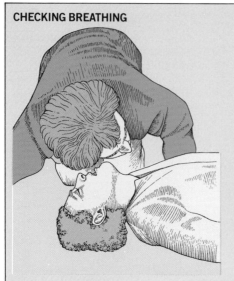

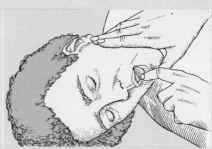

Check his breathing by putting your ear against his nose or mouth, and look along his chest. He is breathing if you can feel breaths against your face and/or see his chest moving.

If he is not breathing
There may be something blocking his air passages — a piece of food or a broken tooth, for example — turn his head to one side and sweep round the inside of his mouth with your finger. Lift out anything you find and check his breathing again. If he is still not breathing, begin mouth-to-mouth ventilation, see opposite.

If he is breathing
■ Loosen his clothing at the neck and chest.
■ Put him in the recovery position (see below).
■ Stay with him all the time and watch to make sure that he does not stop breathing — so long as he is breathing his heart will be beating.

RECOVERY POSITION

This position keeps the tongue forward and the mouth low so that the airway is kept clear and the patient can breathe easily.

1 Turn the person's head to one side and tilt his head back as far as possible.

2 Place his nearest arm by his side and, keeping his hand flat, slide it underneath his buttock; it may be necessary to lift his buttock

slightly. Bring his other arm up and lay it across his chest. Raise the ankle of the leg furthest from you and cross it over his near one.

3 Kneel beside the patient, level with his chest, support his head with one hand and grasp the clothing at the hip furthest from you. Pull him towards you until he is resting against your knees.

4 Re-adjust his head so that it is tilted as far back as possible. Then, bend his uppermost arm and leg and position them so that he cannot roll on to his face.

5 Make sure his other arm is completely free. If it is not, ease it away from his back and leave it lying parallel to it.

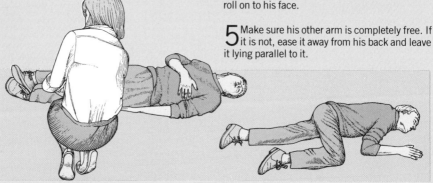

If the person is not breathing
START MOUTH-TO-MOUTH VENTILATION
IMMEDIATELY

MOUTH-TO-MOUTH VENTILATION

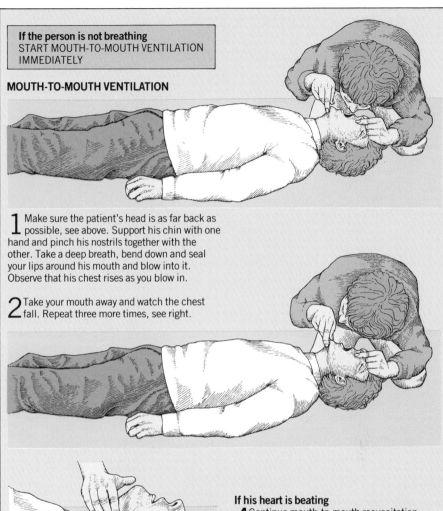

1 Make sure the patient's head is as far back as possible, see above. Support his chin with one hand and pinch his nostrils together with the other. Take a deep breath, bend down and seal your lips around his mouth and blow into it. Observe that his chest rises as you blow in.

2 Take your mouth away and watch the chest fall. Repeat three more times, see right.

3 Check the carotid pulse (the pulse in his neck) to see if the heart is beating. Put two fingers in the groove at the side of his Adam's apple and press firmly. This pulse is used because it is the one nearest to the heart.

If his heart is beating
4 Continue mouth-to-mouth resuscitation, giving 16-18 breaths per minute until he starts breathing again. When he does start breathing again, turn him over into the recovery position, see opposite. Stay with him, watching his breathing all the time, until medical help arrives. Re-start mouth-to-mouth if he stops breathing again.

If his heart is not beating
START CHEST COMPRESSION
IMMEDIATELY, see overleaf.

CHEST COMPRESSION

1 Lay the patient on his back on the floor or other firm surface and kneel alongside him. Find the centre of the breastbone (the bone that runs down the centre of the chest) by measuring with both hands as shown. Put the heel of one hand on the lower half and cover it with the heel of the other hand (see inset).

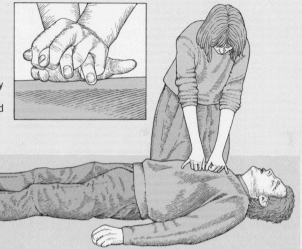

2 Keeping your arm as straight as you can, press down hard on the lower half of the breast-bone to a depth of about 4-5cm (1½-2in) then release the pressure. Continue pressing at a rate of 70-80 times a minute. To help keep time, count out the rhythm "one-and-two-and-three-" and so on, see right.

3 After pressing 15 times, give two quick breaths of mouth-to-mouth ventilation as described on page 103. Continue giving 15 compressions and two breaths in this way.

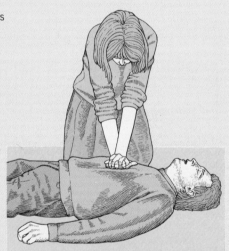

4 After one minute, check the carotid pulse again to see if the heart has started beating. If it is still not beating, continue giving 15 compressions followed by two breaths of mouth-to-mouth stopping every three minutes to check the pulse, until the heart starts beating.

5 Once the heart has started beating, continue with mouth-to-mouth on its own until the patient starts breathing on his own again.

6 Once he has started breathing, put him in the recovery position and wait for medical help to arrive. Stay with the person, watching him all the time as he is liable to stop breathing and his heart may stop beating again. If he stops breathing again you must restart mouth-to-mouth and, if necessary, chest compression.

WARNING

Do not attempt chest compression if the heart is beating even faintly. You can easily disrupt the rhythm and cause it to stop. Equally, you should *never* practise chest compression on anyone whose heart is beating.

HOME OR HOSPITAL?

In the 1960s and 1970s sophisticated monitoring equipment was introduced which can recognize any deterioration in the heart's function the moment it develops, and special Coronary Care Units (CCU) were set up in many hospitals, staffed by highly skilled doctors and nurses. It was thought that early recognition and treatment of complications would save thousands of lives.

Within a decade or so, however, some of the drawbacks had become apparent. First of all, it was realized that life-threatening complications usually occur within the first couple of hours after a heart attack, but that the interval between the heart attack occurring, the patient or relative calling for medical help, and actual admission to a CCU is often longer than that, which means that several lives are lost that could otherwise be saved. Secondly, some people are so intimidated by the CCU's electronic gadgets, that some of the unit's advantages are wiped out.

If your general practitioner is prepared to visit you as frequently as necessary, if there are no complications, if your general health is otherwise good, and if you have a capable partner or relatives who are willing to nurse you during your recovery, there is no reason why you should not stay at home, surrounded by the warmth and loving care of your family. It is quite likely, though, that anxiety on your part and that of a partner and relatives, who feel uneasy about your safety, coupled with the professional concern of your doctor who does not want to take any risk, will result in your being transferred to hospital and preferably a coronary care unit.

YOUR STAY IN HOSPITAL

What happens during your stay in hospital varies from patient to patient. You may feel perfectly well, the chest pain which sent you to hospital in the first place may disappear before you even arrive, and you may simply feel irritated at being there and want to go home. You may, on the other hand, experience recurring episodes of chest pain, weakness, shortness of breath or other complications. Thus you may find yourself wondering what is wrong with you and what is going to happen to you. Alternatively, you may be critically ill and surrounded by such a flurry of activity that you think you will die.

However you feel, it is vitally important not to panic: this makes matters worse. Stress hormones which are released during panic can cause a serious type of rhythm disturbance which can sometimes result in heart failure.

THE CORONARY CARE UNIT

First of all you will probably be admitted to the coronary care unit, a specially equipped hospital unit, where nurses and doctors are all trained in heart disease. The coronary care nurse, even if he or she is not visible to you, will be watching you constantly. The nurse monitors all the vital signs, administers medications prescribed, watches for any adverse physical or psychological reactions, and tries to alleviate them, if necessary with the help of the other members of the team. A doctor does not usually remain with you all the time, however he will never be far away and can be summoned at a moment's notice.

EQUIPMENT IN THE CORONARY CARE UNIT

Coronary care units (CCUs) are equipped for maximum observation and care. There will be monitoring equipment near your bed which records information about your heart's activity and other bodily functions and, in most hospitals, this is also relayed to the CCU's nursing station, which is under 24-hour surveillance. Any irregularities will cause an alarm bell to ring in the nursing station. Not all irregularities are serious, however, so you need not be frightened by the alarm bell. In some hospitals, the CCU has a closed circuit TV transmitting to the nursing station.

Nursing station

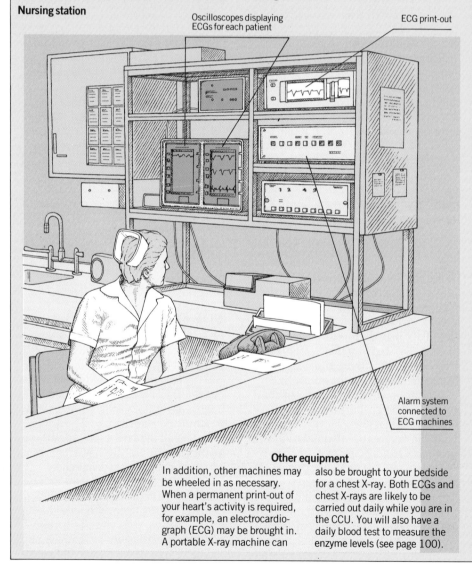

Oscilloscopes displaying ECGs for each patient

ECG print-out

Alarm system connected to ECG machines

Other equipment

In addition, other machines may be wheeled in as necessary. When a permanent print-out of your heart's activity is required, for example, an electrocardiograph (ECG) may be brought in. A portable X-ray machine can also be brought to your bedside for a chest X-ray. Both ECGs and chest X-rays are likely to be carried out daily while you are in the CCU. You will also have a daily blood test to measure the enzyme levels (see page 100).

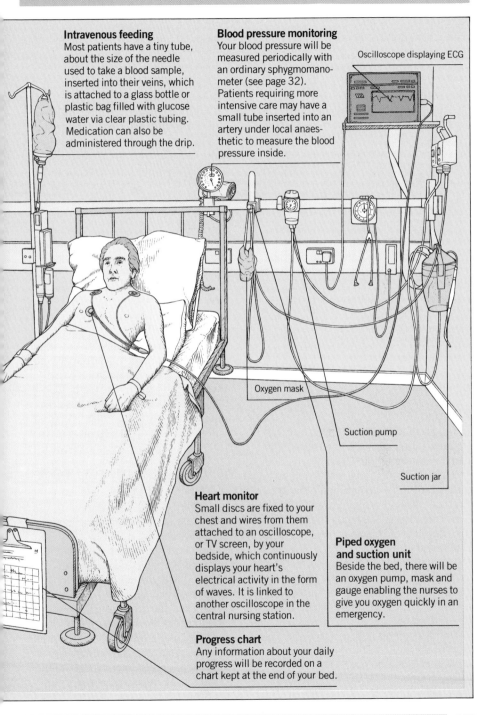

Intravenous feeding
Most patients have a tiny tube, about the size of the needle used to take a blood sample, inserted into their veins, which is attached to a glass bottle or plastic bag filled with glucose water via clear plastic tubing. Medication can also be administered through the drip.

Blood pressure monitoring
Your blood pressure will be measured periodically with an ordinary sphygmomano-meter (see page 32). Patients requiring more intensive care may have a small tube inserted into an artery under local anaes-thetic to measure the blood pressure inside.

Oscilloscope displaying ECG

Oxygen mask

Suction pump

Suction jar

Heart monitor
Small discs are fixed to your chest and wires from them attached to an oscilloscope, or TV screen, by your bedside, which continuously displays your heart's electrical activity in the form of waves. It is linked to another oscilloscope in the central nursing station.

Piped oxygen and suction unit
Beside the bed, there will be an oxygen pump, mask and gauge enabling the nurses to give you oxygen quickly in an emergency.

Progress chart
Any information about your daily progress will be recorded on a chart kept at the end of your bed.

The medical team

A junior house doctor who undertakes most of the day-to-day duties will visit you several times a day and ask relevant medical questions, examine you, set up a lot of monitoring instruments, and answer any query you or your family may have. He will also carry out, or order to be carried out, several tests. Next in the hierarchy is the registrar who will visit you at least once a day, or more often if necessary. The consultant, the head of the team, does not visit daily but will be regularly informed of your condition and is consulted whenever his opinion is needed.

Other members of the team are the physiotherapist, occupational therapist, dietician, psychiatrist or psychologist, radiographer and laboratory technicians. A clergyman or the hospital chaplain is also at hand to counsel you on spiritual matters. The combined function of the team members is to help you recover from your heart attack as smoothly as possible.

Bed rest

In the first few days and especially the first few hours after a heart attack, the damaged heart is particularly sensitive, and any undue activity may bring on an undesirable change in blood pressure or heart rhythm, chest pain or other problems concerning the heart's functioning. Because of this, complete bed rest is necessary and, if you are feeling restless, sedatives or sleeping pills may be prescribed. You will also be given a strong painkiller, usually by injection, to relieve your chest pain, which may be quite severe.

You will spend between two and four days in the CCU but if there are any complications (see page 110), you may be there longer. For the first couple of days you will not be allowed out of bed,

to shave, wash or even go to the toilet. A commode will be brought to your bedside. You will be fed semi-solids and a physiotherapist will move your arms and legs for you to encourage the peripheral circulation.

If your heart attack is mild and there are no complications, you may not have any other treatment. You will be closely monitored and additional treatment may be given only if complications are expected or have already occurred. In some hospitals, anticoagulants (which thin the blood) or fibrinolytic drugs (which dissolve a blood clot) may be given, although the benefits of these drugs are still being reviewed. The drugs are administered intravenously for the first couple of days. Thereafter anticoagulant drugs taken by mouth will be continued for six to eight weeks or, rarely, for even longer.

By the second or third day you may be encouraged to move your arms and legs yourself, to wash your face and hands, and to brush your teeth. The head of your bed will be raised so that you are nearly sitting up, and you may be allowed to sit up in a chair. You may by now also watch television or read.

MOVING OUT OF CCU TO A GENERAL WARD

After two to four days, when you require less intensive monitoring and emergency treatment but more active recovery and rehabilitation, you will be transferred to a general ward. You will stay here until you are discharged – usually between 10 and 14 days after you suffered the heart attack.

In charge of the nurses on the ward is a staff nurse or a ward sister. His or her function is to nurse you, administer medications, record your pulse, blood pressure and temperature, report on your progress to the doctors, and detect any physical or psychological distress. The doctors will also visit you every day, examine your heart and chest, and probably check your carotid pulse (the artery in your neck, see page 19) to monitor the pumping strength of the heart. They will study the pulse and blood pressure charts and the results of blood tests, ECG and chest X-rays, prescribe any drugs you need and generally monitor your progress.

While you are in this ward, you will be asked to start walking and to exercise your limbs while standing. Instead of a commode you will be allowed to use the toilet and you will gradually advance from washing and sponging yourself down to taking a shower or bath.

A physiotherapist will instruct you in the simple exercise of your limbs. You will be asked, to begin with, to walk about in the ward and a few days later in the hospital corridors. You will also be encouraged to climb a few steps, and before you leave the hospital you will be managing short flights of stairs. The physiotherapist will also advise you on a graded exercise programme which you should follow when you go home. You will be advised to spread out your activities and exercises as much as possible after you are discharged from hospital so that you do not tire yourself out and put your heart under too much strain.

Your diet will progress from semi-solids to light meals and just before you leave hospital you will be eating normal food. A dietician will explain that eating habits may have contributed to your heart attack and could still aggravate your condition. You will be advised on safe foods, those that should be eaten only in moderation, and those that are best avoided. Healthy food need not be boring and the dietician can direct you and your partner to attractive and satisfying menus.

The occupational therapist can show you how to cope with activities at home once you are discharged: how to bathe, dress and undress, while imposing the least strain on your heart. You will be advised when you will be able to carry out more strenuous tasks such as cooking or light gardening and other household jobs. The occupational therapist will also visit you in the ward to make sure that you do not get bored while you are in hospital.

You will be given a lot of advice during your hospital stay about diet, exercise, medications, what activities to avoid and so on, and you may end up feeling confused and anxious because you can't remember everything you've been told. This is where this book will come in: you can use it as a reference source to help you along the road to recovery and prevent any further recurrence. More of what you can do yourself is in the self-help section, see pages 124 to 186. However, do not forget that if you are worried, you can always ask your doctor for any advice and he can put you in touch with dieticians and other therapists outside the hospital.

YOUR EMOTIONAL STATE
In the concern for your immediate physical needs, your emotional problems may be overlooked by the medical staff and by your family. You will almost certainly feel anxious, and fears, worries and questions will probably flood into your mind. Will I die? What will happen to my family? Will I become an invalid? Will I be able to return to work and lead a normal life? You may become confused because you do not understand what is happening to you; perhaps the information you have been given is either inadequate or so profuse and technical that it makes no sense. Your anxiety may manifest itself

in restlessness, frustration, insomnia, arguments or even bursts of anger.

In response to your heart attack, you may feel sad, lose interest in things, and experience feelings of withdrawal, hopelessness and dread. Mild depression of this kind is not uncommon. Once you accept this, you will probably be able to handle it without any difficulty. Severe depression, on the other hand, can hinder your recovery and may require both medication and psychological counselling. The hospital staff are trained to recognize depression.

If you feel anxious, withdrawn and depressed while you are in hospital, you may be asked to see a psychologist or social worker. If your spirits are low and you've reached the point where you doubt whether life is worth living, remember that a hospital chaplain or priest is also available to counsel you, and you should not hesitate to seek help.

TESTS BEFORE DISCHARGE

In addition to routine and frequent ECGs, chest X-rays and blood tests, you may also have one of the tests outlined in Chapter 8 (see pages 86 to 90).

In particular, you are likely to have a low level exercise stress test on a stationary bicycle or treadmill, which can help in the planning of your activities after you have been discharged (see page 120). A heart scan can not only confirm the diagnosis of a heart attack but can also tell the extent of the damage and the pumping strength of the heart (see page 89). Holter monitoring can detect intermittent rhythm disturbances, which may explain bouts of dizzy spells or fainting attacks (see page 88).

If you continue to have angina, you can have a cardiac catheterization and coronary angiogram, which can detect the location and degree of narrowing, the size of the damage, the likelihood of future attacks, and the overall strength of the heart muscle (see page 89). These tests are invariably carried out before bypass surgery is considered (see page 93). The operation may be delayed for a few weeks after a heart attack, in which case you will be discharged from hospital after ten to 14 days, and then readmitted later.

POSSIBLE COMPLICATIONS

By and large, serious complications after a heart attack are rare and 80 per cent of patients admitted to a CCU recover completely. Described here are some of the complications that occur in a very small percentage of patients.

Heart rhythm disturbance

Even before your heart attack, you may have been aware of your heart beats, or you may have experienced a feeling of missed beats (palpitations), particularly after too much coffee or alcohol or too many cigarettes. The odd missed beat is not abnormal and is not a cause for concern. You may also have been aware of rapid heart beats after strenuous activity or emotional stress.

A heart attack patient is especially prone to heart rhythm disturbances. These fall into three categories:

- Slower than normal heart rate (bradycardia)
- Faster than normal heart rate (tachycardia)
- Irregular rhythm (arrythmia) ranging from simple premature (or missed) beats to more serious flutter, or fibrillation, of either upper or lower chambers of the heart.

A serious rhythm disturbance undermines the pumping action of the heart and interferes with the blood supply to both the brain and coronary arteries, causing dizziness, fainting or angina; it needs urgent treatment.

If premature beats (often known as missed beats because there is a long interval between the premature beat and the resumption of normal heart beats) occur frequently, drugs may be given to suppress the heart's "irritability" and to prevent serious arrythmia. Lidocaine (Xylocaine) is usually given by intravenous injection. Some hospitals give this drug routinely to *prevent* arrhythmia, even if the heart is beating regularly.

If the heart is beating too quickly, beta-blockers may be given by injection. Other drugs used are procainamide, quinidine or digoxin. If the heart is beating too slowly, you may feel faint or dizzy. Atropine or isoprenaline may be given by injection. If it continues to beat slowly, an artificial pacemaker will be fitted, to stimulate the heart muscle electrically (see page 116).

If one of the most serious types of rhythm disturbance has developed in which the heart is not beating but only quivering (known as fibrillation), then immediate electric stimulation (defibrillation) is given. This often succeeds in jolting the fluttering, or quivering, heart back into a normally beating one.

CCUs are so well equipped that there is hardly any rhythm disturbance that cannot be treated successfully. Rhythm-suppressing drugs sometimes have to be continued even after you have been discharged from hospital.

Congestive heart failure

The term heart failure is both frightening and misleading. In heart failure, the heart is weakened and so its pumping function becomes less efficient. As a result, less blood is pumped into the body, which can lead to congested lungs, shortness of breath and fluid retention, the most common manifestations of which are swollen ankles and, less comonly, legs and abdomen. Heart failure can also occur without a heart attack, in which case its onset is more gradual.

Treatment consists of digoxin tablets, which increase the strength of contraction of the heart muscle and also slow down the rate of heart beats, and diuretics, or water pills, which help to remove excess water and salt from the body through increased urination. Other drugs may also be used if there is associated high blood pressure or angina. The heart can regain its power with appropriate treatment, though it is likely that treatment may have to continue for a long time, sometimes for ever.

Cardiac shock

The word shock is used by lay people in a number of different ways, but doctors define the term for medical purposes as a condition in which the flow of blood throughout the body suddenly becomes inadequate. This may occur after a heart attack if the heart's pumping action is suddenly and drastically impaired so that it pumps out an inadequate supply of blood. Lack of blood to the brain may affect the nervous control of the blood vessels in the body, particularly in the stomach area. The vessel walls become floppy and the space within them is increased. A large amount of blood collects in them and blood pressure plummets to an unacceptably low level. Once the downward spiral begins, immediate treatment is essential; untreated shock will result in death.

Symptoms include sweating, faintness, nausea, breathlessness and a rapid but weak pulse. The patient may look pale, with cold and clammy hands, the pulse is rapid and weak and blood pressure may be too low to measure. As the blood supply to the brain falls, a person in shock becomes drowsy, confused, and may even lose consciousness.

Treatment entails pumping blood or plasma into the circulation. Oxygen may also be given, as well as drugs to raise blood pressure.

Deep-vein thrombosis

One of the possible complications of bed rest is deep-vein thrombosis, which affects three to four per cent of heart attack patients. When the circulation of the blood becomes sluggish, a blood clot (thrombus) forms in a vein, usually in the legs. This is more likely to happen if you are overweight and old. Thrombosis in a leg causes swelling and pain in the affected area, but if the clot occurs elsewhere in the body, there may be no symptoms at all unless a large piece (embolus) breaks off and is swept away into the circulation and lodges in a vein within the lungs. This condition, called pulmonary embolism, leads to faintness, shortness of breath and chest pain, and may cause the patient to cough up blood-stained sputum. If an embolus is massive, the patient may collapse and die.

The best way to prevent deep-vein thrombosis is by encouraging the movement of the limbs during a period of bed

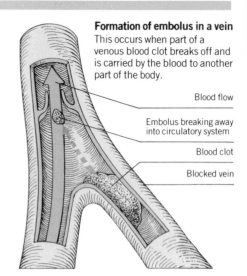

Formation of embolus in a vein
This occurs when part of a venous blood clot breaks off and is carried by the blood to another part of the body.

Blood flow

Embolus breaking away into circulatory system

Blood clot

Blocked vein

rest – so physiotherapy is crucial. If thrombosis has already occurred, you may be given anticoagulants to thin the blood. In difficult cases, drugs that dissolve clots may be injected; surgical removal of the thrombus or embolus is sometimes necessary.

Heart aneurysm

Before the scar tissue has replaced the damaged muscle, the wall of the heart is weak. If blood pressure is too high, or if too much activity is undertaken too soon, or sometimes for no apparent reason, there can be a ballooning of the heart wall called an aneurysm. This is a very rare complication indeed and is very serious if it develops.

DRUGS AFTER DISCHARGE

If you have suffered a mild heart attack, it is quite possible that you will be discharged without any drugs, and with only advice on diet, exercise and rest. On the other hand, there may have been a slight complication that your doctor wants to treat with drugs, in which case,

you may be prescribed one of the drugs described on the following pages.

Anticoagulants

These drugs thin the blood and, at least in theory, prevent further thrombosis either in the veins or in the coronary arteries; they may be given for a few weeks or months. They will normally be given to prevent deep-vein thrombosis in the legs. Unfortunately, however, they do not always succeed in preventing a further heart attack. The disadvantages are that you are required to have frequent blood tests – maybe as often as two or three times a week to start with and then at weekly intervals. If you are on long-term anticoagulants, you will have a blood test once a month after the first few weeks of stabilization. A possible danger is that of serious bruises and internal or external bleeding if the blood is thinned too much.

The most commonly prescribed anticoagulant is coumarin (trade name, Warfarin). If you are prescribed an anticoagulant, you must not take any other drugs without consulting your doctor.

Anti-thrombotic drugs
Aspirin and/or other drugs, such as persantin, which reduce the stickiness of blood platelets and thus the tendency for the blood to coagulate, may also be prescribed.

The advantages of this kind of treatment for heart attack patients are not, as yet, very clear and there may be problems of gastro-intestinal upsets and, less commonly, the formation of stomach ulcers and internal bleeding. Aspirin is never prescribed with Warfarin because the two drugs can react with each other, causing internal or external bleeding.

OTHER DRUGS
The other types of treatment which may be prescribed are those for angina (see Chapter 8), heart failure (page 111), rhythm disturbance (page 110), and high blood pressure (Chapter 7) and those prescribed in the hope of preventing a further heart attack. These medications are all long term, sometimes for

the rest of your life and it is essential that you know exactly what their purpose is, how much and how often they have to be taken and in what quantity, and for how long they are to continue. It is important that you raise this last point with your doctor from time to time. Although you must continue to take your drugs exactly as they have been prescribed for you, you must also realize that they are not the be all and end all: what they can do is limited and the self-help measures which are described in Chapters 10 to 14 are probably just as – if not more – important.

Anti-hypertensives
The drugs used to control high blood pressure are discussed in Chapter 7. There is no conclusive evidence that they prevent further heart attacks and they may not be without their dangers. In a large trial in the United States called MRFIT (Multiple Risk Factor Intervention Trial), it was shown that among those people with ECG abnormality at the start of the trial, more died in the group who were on drugs for high blood pressure than in the group who were not on such medications.

Blood-fat reducing drugs
Since a raised level of fats in the blood is associated with an increased chance of having a heart attack, it follows that drugs that can reduce fat levels are used in the hope of preventing a recurrence. It should be remembered, though, that the first step is to make every effort to reduce fat levels by changing to a diet low in saturated and high in polyunsaturated fats (see page 128). The drugs will be given only if the levels remain dangerously high.

One such drug, in use for several years, was Clofibrate; then an international trial was carried out to see if its use could be further extended to healthy people with raised blood cholesterol levels. Fifteen thousand people from Edinburgh, Budapest and Prague took part and, after five years, some rather surprising truths were revealed: the drug certainly reduced the risk of having a heart attack, but, overall, it killed more people than it saved. Most of these deaths were from diseases of the gall bladder, liver and bowel, including cancer. The trial was described in the medical journal *The Lancet* thus: "The treatment was beneficial but the patient died!" The drug is no longer in use.

There are other drugs which can reduce fat levels in the blood. It is true that they may reduce the chances of future heart attacks, but their benefits are not impressive and are likely to be wiped out by their side-effects. In 1985, two scientists, Doctor Joseph Goldstein and Doctor Michael Brown, won the Nobel prize for their research on the structure and function of an enzyme whose activity is vital in the synthesis of cholesterol by the body. This gives new hope that one day soon researchers will find a new drug that will block production of cholesterol by the body.

Beta-blockers

There has recently been a tendency for some doctors to prescribe long-term beta-blockers to prevent a recurrence. They may be useful for some people but their wholesale use is to be discouraged for the following reasons. In the first place, they can cause a number of side-effects, including wheeziness, fatigue, depression, weight gain, hallucinations, nightmares, insomnia, cold extremities and psoriasis-like skin rashes.

Secondly, they may interfere with your self-healing ability by masking physical warning signs and emotional over-arousal. Thirdly, you may come to rely on them to such an extent that those problems that may have caused the heart attack in the first place are pushed to one side and remain unresolved. In addition, they tend to have an adverse effect on the level of blood fats and so tend to counteract some of their benefits. And finally, their benefits may not last longer than one year. These drugs are described in detail in Chapter 7.

If you have been prescribed them, however, you must continue to take them regularly as an abrupt stoppage can have serious or even fatal results.

SURGICAL TREATMENT

If drug treatment fails to relieve you of angina or if you are believed to be at risk of further heart damage, you may be recommended to have a coronary bypass operation. This is discussed in detail in Chapter 8 on angina. Other possible surgical treatment includes a heart transplant (see opposite) or the use of an artificial pacemaker.

PACEMAKERS

The treatment of patients who have an abnormally slow heartbeat with artificial pacemakers has transformed a short inactive life, declining to an early death within a few months of the appearance of the disease, to an active life that can continue for many years.

The heart's own pacemaker

Your heart performs the mechanical task of pumping blood around the body but, like any machine, it needs a power supply – the electrical impulses which stimulate the heart muscle to contract. These impulses are normally controlled by the heart's natural pacemaker, a microscopic structure called the sino-atrial node, which is situated in the upper left chamber of the heart and produces some 72 impulses a minute while the body is resting (see page 14).

If the heart pacemaker fails

Faults can develop in the complex electrical conducting system of the heart. The sinoatrial node may become unreliable and may either cease sending impulses altogether or produce only intermittent impulses. This is called sinoatrial node disease and may occur as part of the ageing process, or as a result of heart disease, heart attack or surgery. When the impulses fail to reach the

ventricles, or reach them irregularly, this condition is called heart block, which may be complete or partial.

Signs and symptoms

The result of heart block is an extremely slow heart rate because the ventricles can contract only through their own spontaneous rhythm at the rate of 40 beats or less per minute, irrespective of demand. If the demands on the heart are increased, it becomes less efficient as a pumping organ; if increased demand continues, heart failure occurs. Sometimes the heart may stop altogether, leading to temporary unconsciousness. This may occur without any warning, or after a bout of unexplained dizzy spells.

HEART TRANSPLANT

This is the most extreme form of surgery carried out to help patients with heart disease. If the function of the heart muscle is so weakened that the pumping chambers are not able to pump out more than 30 per cent of the blood they receive, a heart transplant is considered. In many heart transplant operations, the surgeon does not actually remove the entire heart, but cuts away only the two main pumping chambers

(ventricles), the main heart valves and part of the two upper chambers (atria). Most of the major blood vessels remain, to which the donor's heart is then sewn.

The main problem involved in heart (and other) transplants is the body's rejection of foreign tissue. A number of drugs that suppress the rejection process have been developed and, as a result, an increasing number of transplants are now successful.

What the operation entails

An incision will be made down the centre of your breastbone, and you will be connected up to a

heart/lung machine. Most of your heart will be removed and the donor heart will be sewn on to the remaining part of your own heart.

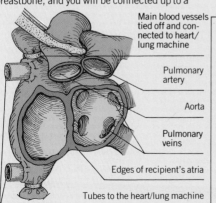

Main blood vessels tied off and connected to heart/lung machine

Pulmonary artery

Aorta

Pulmonary veins

Edges of recipient's atria

Tubes to the heart/lung machine

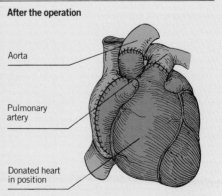

After the operation

Aorta

Pulmonary artery

Donated heart in position

In many patients with complete heart block and sinoatrial node disease, the heart is otherwise normal. If an artificial pacemaker is successfully implanted, the performance of the heart can be restored virtually to normal and the person can resume an active life.

Temporary problems

After a heart attack, a disturbance may occur in the heart's electrical system which eventually corrects itself as you recover. Implantation of a temporary artificial pacemaker during the early days of recovery may be life-saving.

ARTIFICIAL PACEMAKERS

A pacemaker can provide a complete cure for the heart's electrical defects and, provided you do not suffer from any other diseases of the heart and your device is checked regularly, you can forget about your pacemaker and enjoy life to the full. A pacemaking system consists of an electrical pulse generator connected to an electrode by one or two wires. The pulse generator is about the size of a matchbox, weighs 50-100g (2-4oz), and consists of two parts – the power supply, or batteries, and the electronic circuitry (see opposite). Electrical impulses generated by the small pulse generator are carried via the wires to the electrode which is situated in the heart to stimulate its contraction and so produce a heart beat. The entire system is sealed in a metal casing to prevent body fluids from seeping into the unit.

Most pacemakers fall into one of these two categories:
- External pacemakers, for temporary use only
- Implanted, permanent pacemakers.

External pacemakers

These are used for temporary pacing while a patient is in hospital and are always removed when they are no longer needed: in patients who develop rhythm disturbance after a heart attack or open heart surgery, for example, but regain normal function as they recover; or as an emergency measure before fitting a permanent pacemaker. The generating unit is either strapped to the body or worn on a belt or around the neck.

Implanted pacemakers

When a permanent pacemaker is required, the generating unit is implanted in the body. Modern pacemakers can be as small as 1cm ($\frac{1}{2}$in) thick and 4cm ($1\frac{1}{2}$in) wide and weigh just over 40g ($1\frac{1}{2}$oz). The majority are powered by lithium batteries, which can last between five and 12 years depending on the size of the battery or the type of pacemaker used.

Implanted pacemakers may be either insensitive or sensitive to the natural heart rhythm. A fixed-rate pacemaker is insensitive, completely ignoring the natural rhythm of the heart and discharging at a pre-set rate. It is used when the heart rate is permanently slow. A demand pacemaker is sensitive to the natural heart beat: each time the heart beats, the pacemaker's electrical impulse is suppressed; but every time the heart misses a beat, the pacemaker's electrical impulse is discharged. Most pacemakers are of the demand variety.

There is a third type of pacemaker which can be programmed to work either at a fixed rate or on demand, according to a patient's changing needs. The programme can be altered externally, by means of electromagnetic signals, even after the pacemaker has been implanted. Some pacemakers automatically change their discharge rate without external programming. These physiological pacemakers are more complex and often have two

PACEMAKERS

There is very little difference in the outward appearance of the different pacemakers. Some have one electrode lead attached to one part of the heart, others have two electrodes, one leading to the upper chamber and one to the lower chamber.

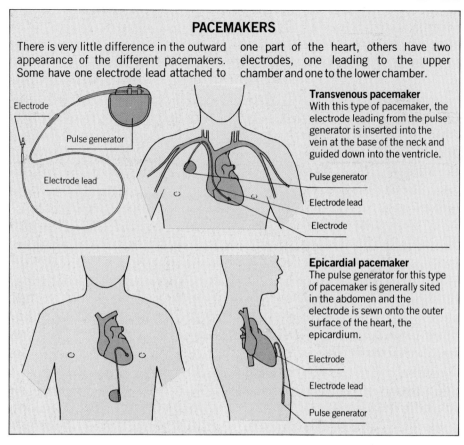

Transvenous pacemaker
With this type of pacemaker, the electrode leading from the pulse generator is inserted into the vein at the base of the neck and guided down into the ventricle.

Pulse generator

Electrode lead

Electrode

Electrode

Pulse generator

Electrode lead

Epicardial pacemaker
The pulse generator for this type of pacemaker is generally sited in the abdomen and the electrode is sewn onto the outer surface of the heart, the epicardium.

Electrode

Electrode lead

Pulse generator

electrode leads implanted in the upper and lower chambers of the heart, which are stimulated in sequence to restore the normal function of the heart.

Another type of pacemaker that is being used now interrupts or prevents fast heart rates and analyses information about the natural heart rhythm.

Pacemaker implantation

This is generally carried out in the X-ray department, where you lie flat on your back with the X-ray machinery above your chest. The main techniques are transvenous and epicardial.

The transvenous method entails a hospital stay of two or three days. The electrode is inserted, under local anaesthetic, into a vein near the base of the neck. It is guided, with the help of X-rays, into the right ventricle and an ECG is recorded from inside the heart to establish when the electrode is firmly secured in a stable position. The free end is connected to the pulse generator, which is then implanted just beneath the collarbone in a pocket made under the skin. The whole procedure takes less than an hour.

In the epicardial method, a general anaesthetic is usual and you are likely to be in hospital for about five or six days. The electrode is introduced through a small incision just below the breastbone and attached to the outside of the heart wall (epicardium), while the pulse generator is buried in the abdominal wall.

Follow-up treatment

In the early stages after having a pacemaker fitted, you will attend the pacemaker clinic at frequent intervals – say, a month after discharge and again at the end of a further three months. Thereafter a regular six-monthly check is usual. The pacemaker's rate is tested electronically and the device is replaced well before the batteries run out.

Obviously, if a major fault develops suddenly, your original symptoms will develop (dizziness or blackouts) and you must contact your doctor or clinic immediately. It is wise to carry a medical card at all times, giving essential details about yourself, your cardiac condition and your pacemaker so that, in the unlikely event of your needing emergency treatment, the doctor will have all the details he needs to help you.

Electromagnetic interference

Fixed-rate pacemakers do not contain any sensing circuits and are influenced neither by biological signals nor by outside electromagnetic interference. A demand pacemaker, however, has to be sensitive to the natural heart rhythm and contains sensing circuits. External electromagnetic signals, some of which closely mimic the heart's own signal, may therefore suppress the pacemaker's electrical impulse.

In practice this rarely happens, since the pacemakers are well shielded from such signals, but in theory at least, spot-welding machines, anti-theft devices, metal detectors, electromagnets, radio and TV transmitters, metal detectors used in airports and libraries, and faulty microwave ovens can all occasionally influence the working of a pacemaker. Manufacturers of pacemakers give detailed instructions as to exactly which sources of electromagnetic interference must be avoided.

CARING FOR THE PATIENT AT HOME

When someone you love has a heart attack, the experience can be alarming, confusing and emotionally draining. Many of the financial, psychological and social problems that both you and the patient are likely to face can be resolved, or at least their burden can be reduced, if you can learn to share them between you and to discuss them openly and constructively with each other. You can also help the patient to recover by maintaining a positive, cheerful and optimistic attitude. Discuss the information you and the patient are given and plan a sensible programme of rehabilitation.

It is particularly important that you appreciate the difference between instructions you are given which are merely intended as guidelines, and those which must be adhered to strictly. Advice regarding medication must be strictly followed, but some of the other recommendations can be given greater latitude. There is nothing more annoying for a patient than your trying to follow every piece of advice you have been given to the letter – by throwing away favourite foods, recording every sip of alcohol, or timing every minute's exercise with a stopwatch.

Let the patient know his recovery is important to you and that you are there to assist in every possible way. Offer sympathy and understanding but don't take over his life completely. Many people are proud, and their ego is wounded if you appear to cope too adequately without them, so be as tactful as you can. Share your interests and hobbies with the patient, so that he does not feel isolated and, most important of all, plan a realistic future and work towards this goal together.

Anxiety and depression

It is natural for someone who has had a heart attack to worry about the future – returning to work, possible financial problems, relationships with partner and family members, social standing, changes in future plans, and so on – but all these anxieties can be resolved, to a large extent, by mutual discussion. If they are not managed properly right from the start, they can lead to irritability, arguments and insomnia, all of which can hinder recovery. It is most important to help the patient accept that he has not been singled out for this personal tragedy and it is possible to make the necessary adjustments with patience and understanding and, if you need expert advice, you can get guidance from professional people.

It is not unusual for a patient to withdraw, to feel sad, to shed tears, and to lose interest in everything. Neither is it unreasonable for him to have such reactions when he has just had to face a serious, life-threatening situation, after which the future seems depressingly uncertain. He may feel particularly frustrated at having to take things easy and not being able to do everything as quickly and easily as before.

Occasionally, in spite of recovery from a heart attack, a patient may continue to complain that he has no energy and, even several months after returning to work, may remain as distant as in the early days after the attack. In such difficult cases, drugs and/or psychotherapy may be required.

Denial

The refusal to believe that he has just suffered a heart attack is quite common among heart attack victims. While it pushes away the painful reality – and this can be useful in a moment of crisis – it also interferes with the recovery programme and prevents a patient from seeking medical advice whenever necessary. If someone close to you has had a heart attack, you must help him to come to terms with his condition.

THE ROAD TO RECOVERY

Leaving hospital may cause anxiety and uneasiness both to you and your family. It is easy to be frightened by the sudden absence of constant and watchful attention from trained staff. You may have doubts about monitoring your exercise, watching your diet, going about your domestic or personal chores and returning to work. You will probably also want to know whether it is safe for you to resume sexual relationships.

Such feelings and concerns are all normal and can be resolved if you keep open the channels of communication with both your family and your doctor. When members of the family make suggestions about diet, exercise, medications or whatever, they are doing so only out of concern for you, and you should work together to re-establish family roles and to resolve conflicts with the minimum possible stress. Try not to forget your sense of humour, and learn to develop an easy, relaxed attitude (see page 150). Your state of mind will affect the speed of your recovery.

ACTIVITY AFTER YOU ARE DISCHARGED

Within just a few days of a heart attack, your innate powers of self-healing are brought into action and you should try to give yourself the best possible chance both to recover and to prevent a recurrence. Over a period of weeks, scar tissue will gradually replace the damaged cells and it is also likely that there will be changes in the blood flow; within two to three weeks of a heart attack, for example, new arteries called collaterals will probably develop around the damaged area in an effort to bring extra blood to the tissues. Physical activities that make you feel slightly out of breath but do not cause angina pain will encourage the development of collaterals. You will therefore be encouraged to increase your activities slowly over the next few months without putting any excessive demands on the heart.

You may feel so well that you want to do more than the schedule that has been suggested to you at the hospital or by your doctor; or you may feel tired and apprehensive that you will not be able to manage as much as you have been recommended. Everyone's recovery rate is different depending on the size of the heart attack, the presence or absence of complications, age, level of fitness before suffering the heart attack, and the body's tolerance to any change in its level of activity.

Return to normality gradually

The important thing is to build up the tasks you set yourself gradually. The same gradual approach applies to exercise. Do not exercise to the point where you become short of breath, tired, dizzy, or suffer from chest pain. If any of these symptoms occurs, stop exercising immediately and rest. If they persist or recur, consult your doctor.

It is quite normal to feel more tired on some days than on others. If you are too tired, wait until the following day before increasing your activities, or even cut down on some of them. Take your time to do each job and don't rush. Alternate a hard task with an easy one and spread out your activities throughout the day. Rest for half an hour once or twice a day, and always rest after meals. If you feel tired, rest for a while and then continue with the activity.

HOW MUCH CAN YOU DO?

In the first two weeks after your discharge from hospital, walk only on the flat, gradually increasing the distance up to 800m ($\frac{1}{2}$ mile). Over the next two weeks increase the distance up to 1200m ($\frac{3}{4}$ mile) and include some steps and walking on a mild incline. Six to eight weeks after the attack, gradually add other activities such as playing a few holes of golf – but don't carry the clubs, use a cart instead. You can also swim, starting with one length, or try a little leisurely cycling. Do a little gardening if you enjoy it – but not heavy digging; and bear in mind that it is better to do two or three periods of ten minutes each than to do half an hour at a stretch.

Carrying things

There is no reason why you can't walk to the neighbourhood shops two to three weeks after the heart attack, provided that you do not carry more than 2.25kg (5lb). In the next couple of weeks, you may double the load up to 4.5kg (10lb), and between six and eight weeks after the attack you may double it again up to 9kg (20lb).

Strenuous exercise

If you really want to do something more strenuous, such as jogging, make sure that you do this under close supervision as it may be inadvisable for you. More competitive sports, such as tennis, should be treated with caution, and squash is best avoided altogether.

The best thing to do is to work out a programme with the help of your doctor or, better still, a sports clinic or gymnasium which specializes in coronary rehabilitation (see page 186).

Sexual activity

For many people, sex is an embarrassing subject that they find difficult to discuss, not only with their doctor but also sometimes with their own partner. It is not surprising, therefore, that many heart attack patients are reluctant to raise the subject. When you can resume sexual activity will depend on how soon you recover your physical strength. If you can manage a brisk walk to cover 275m (300yds) or two flights of stairs without getting breathless or experiencing chest pain, you are ready to resume sexual relations. Most people regain sufficient strength in the heart muscle to cope with the demands of intercourse within six to eight weeks. Remember, though, that this does not preclude physical closeness and intimacy with your partner without actually having intercourse. Avoid having sex after a large meal or if you feel tired.

Driving

Particularly in heavy city traffic, driving can be stressful and can push your blood pressure and heart rate up to quite high levels so you should not drive until your heart has recovered sufficiently. For most people this means waiting for a few months after their heart attack.

Once you have had a heart attack, you will not be allowed to drive public service vehicles or heavy goods vehicles, but there is no reason why you should

not drive your own car. Start with short trips in the neighbourhood and then progress to a longer trip to town before venturing on to a motorway. If you have any doubts, consult your doctor.

OUTINGS AND TRAVEL

Short trips, when you are driven by a friend or a member of your family to go to the theatre, the cinema, or to visit a friend, are usually permissible four weeks after a heart attack. Flying should be avoided for up to six weeks or more, but prior consultation with your doctor is essential as no two patients are alike. You must avoid lifting suitcases and allow plenty of time to handle pre-flight arrangements such as checking in and walking to the aeroplane. Remember, too, that the distance you have to go before boarding the aeroplane can entail quite a long walk and may include a flight of stairs.

FOOD AND DRINK

Eat several small meals a day rather than two or even three large ones. Avoid eating rich fatty foods and eat more fruit and vegetables and wholemeal foods (see also pages 125 to 132). Eat slowly, chew thoroughly and rest after meals.

Limit the amount of coffee you drink to two cups a day as it contains caffeine, which may stimulate or irritate your heart unnecessarily. A small quantity of alcohol – one or two glasses of wine or sherry, if you are used to it – is quite acceptable. You must not drink large amounts – more than 75g (3 floz) in any one day – and never drink enough to get drunk. Alcohol is discussed in greater detail in Chapter 11).

CLIMATE

Avoid extremes of weather. It is best not to participate in outdoor activities when it is really cold – for example, when it is snowing – or when the weather is very hot. It is also advisable to avoid saunas, steam cabinets and hot whirlpool baths.

EMOTIONAL STRAIN

Emotional upsets increase the work your heart has to do, especially if you are also engaged in physical activity. Try to avoid situations that make you angry or upset. If you know that a forthcoming situation is likely to be stressful, and you are unable to avoid it altogether, at least be prepared for it and, if you have them, suck one of your angina tablets beforehand. Learn not to bottle up your emotions but to communicate calmly and effectively. Learn to develop a gentle, relaxed attitude and don't allow yourself to get upset or to be provoked into anger.

STARTING WORK AGAIN

Exactly when you can return depends on the size of your heart attack, any complications, your age and your overall physical and mental health and the nature of your job. It is very important to discuss it with your doctor first.

If your heart attack was a mild, uncomplicated one and your job involved no manual work, there is no reason why you cannot return to work eight weeks after the attack. If, on the other hand, your job involves a lot of responsibility, travel, long hours, heavy manual work or lifting more than 9kg (20lb), it is unwise to return before three months and it may take much longer. It may well be possible to negotiate with your employers to return to lighter work or to work part-time before going back to your usual job.

About 75 per cent of heart attack patients return to work within three months; another 15 per cent return within six months. If you feel that the level of your physical strength does not allow you to do your heavy manual job, discuss this with your doctor. He can help you to register as partially disabled, and a disabled resettlement officer at your local job centre can then help you to find lighter work. About three per cent are able to return to alternative lighter work. Of the seven per cent who do not make it, only half of these fail to do so for medical reasons; the others do not return because of a psychological handicap.

GUIDELINES FOR RECOVERY

● Remain under the supervision of your doctor and specialist. Have regular check-ups and follow their advice.
● If your blood pressure is, or has been, high, you must have it checked regularly and always follow your doctor's advice on its management.
● If you have been prescribed any medication, always take it regularly. Above all, make sure you know what it is for, when it should be taken, and in what quantity. Consult your doctor if you have any side-effects and do not stop taking medication abruptly.
● Stop smoking. A heart patient who continues to smoke 20 cigarettes a day is three times as likely to suffer another heart attack as a non-smoker. One who stops smoking reduces the risk to almost as low as that of people who never smoked. Anti-smoking clinics are often run by hospitals and local health education departments and may help you if you have difficulty in giving up.
● Take care of your general health. Avoid exposure to infection as far as possible and remember to have anti-influenza injections before the winter.
● Watch your diet. Eat a prudent, well-balanced diet which is low in animal fat and cholesterol, high in fresh fruit, vegetables and whole grains. If you become less active, consume fewer

calories to prevent weight gain.
● If you are overweight, reduce your weight gradually, preferably to just below your ideal body weight to give yourself a little leeway (see page 133). Weigh yourself regularly and don't be too ambitious in your weekly target loss.
● Avoid heavy meals. If you eat two big meals a day, switch to four small ones.
● Alcohol is permissible in moderation (a maximum of two standard drinks per day, see page 138) and may even be beneficial to some people. More than two cups of coffee per day may give you heart flutter. Try fruit juice, herb tea and spring water instead.
● Continue to take regular exercise. Walking is good exercise, but running may strain your heart unless you graduate to that level under supervision.
● Avoid any sudden exertion which could bring on angina, such as pushing the car, unjamming a window or carrying a heavy load.
● Avoid exertion in extremes of weather, like walking against cold winds, shovelling snow, or mowing the lawn when it's very hot and humid.
● Adjust to a peaceful but active lifestyle in which you can avoid or control stressful situations as much as possible. Emotional strain can raise your blood pressure and worsen atherosclerosis.
● If you were a workaholic, thriving on continuous challenges and working against hectic deadlines, now is the time to change to a slower pace. Learn to delegate; if possible find some temporary help if you are self-employed.
● Take a few minutes off every couple of hours to relax: remember that relaxation is not a luxury but a necessity. Have a relaxation break instead of a coffee break or business lunch and put away your work while you sip a glass of fruit juice or herbal tea.
● Develop new hobbies.

● Avoid becoming overtired. Don't drive yourself to the point of exhaustion and make sure you have enough sleep.
● Avoid too hectic a social life, with too many parties and late nights.
● Try to maintain a positive outlook on life. Understand what is going on in your heart and take good care of yourself, but don't become neurotic or frightened by your condition.
● Count your blessings instead of your misfortunes. You will be surprised at how many positive things you can find in your life which calm the mind and thus protect your heart.
● Develop feelings of tolerance and consideration for others. If someone is unpleasant to you, instead of getting angry and making yourself miserable, think how bad he must be feeling. Take a few slow, deep breaths; this will calm you down and help you stay in control of your feelings.

CONCLUSION

As I have already explained in Chapters 4 and 5, a heart attack is related to some extent to the way in which you live. The steps you take now that determine your present and future lifestyle may make all the difference between having another heart attack or not. They are much the same as those to prevent coronary heart disease (see Chapters 10 to 14).

Some doctors also claim that the reduction of blood pressure with drugs, and a daily dose of a beta-blocker even if you do not have high blood pressure, can reduce the chances of further heart attacks. While this is true in certain patients, the evidence for its benefit in others is not, as yet, convincing. You should follow your doctor's advice in this matter and, if you have been prescribed medication, you must take it regularly. If you are not happy with your prescription, you must not stop taking it suddenly; consult your doctor.

SELF-HELP SECTION

10
A healthy eating plan

There is much truth in the old saying "You are what you eat", particularly as far as the heart is concerned. Eating the wrong foods increases the risk of heart disease; whereas eating a balanced diet reduces the risk of high blood pressure and atherosclerosis, and can actually protect the cardiovascular system from various diseases. Hence, if you enjoy the right foods and take regular exercise you will be less susceptible to heart or circulatory disease and you will increase your chances of a healthier life.

Over the past twenty years, ideas about which foods are considered to be healthy, and which are not, have altered considerably. Previously it was thought that a good diet involved eating steak,

and other red meats, and cheese and biscuits rather than puddings. It is now realized that these foods contain large proportions of saturated fats and other baddies (see pages 128 to 132). To find out how healthy your diet is, start by examining not just what you eat, but your eating habits in general. When you have read the recommendations in this chapter, you may decide you need to change these habits as well as your diet. If you do, introduce changes gradually so your digestive system can adjust; set yourself weekly targets, as a lifetime's routines and tastes may be difficult to change overnight, though just because food is good for us, it does not mean it is any less diverse or appetizing.

A BALANCED DIET

To achieve a balanced diet you need to include certain amounts of protein, carbohydrate, fats, vitamins and minerals, without which your body is unable to function efficiently, in your intake of food. A mixed and varied diet means that it is almost impossible to go short of any of these requirements, though some cooking methods can affect the vitamin content of certain foods, for

example, vitamin C is destroyed if you boil vegetables for a long time.

The chances are, on the other hand, that you may eat too much fat, particularly saturated fat; too much sugar; too much salt; and not enough fibre. In addition, if you eat more calories (units of food energy), than you burn up, the excess food is deposited as fat and you will gradually become overweight. The problems caused by excess dietary fat, sugar and salt are discussed in greater detail on pages 128 to 132.

You must eat wholefoods

The best way of meeting your body's needs, and thus protecting yourself against heart disease, is to eat a natural wholefood diet and keep processed, or refined, food to a minimum. Processing reduces the nutritional value of many foods and introduces the chemical additives, some of which can have a harmful effect. So, wherever possible, you should eat foods that are as close to their natural state as possible – whole grains and plenty of fresh fruit and vegetables, with their skins where possible, either raw or very lightly cooked.

The importance of fluids

An adequate fluid intake is necessary for the digestion, to regulate body temperature and to flush out waste products. The healthiest drinks are water, fruit juices and vegetable juices. Remember that fruit and vegetables contain water.

Vegetarianism

This is not simply a question of cutting meat out of your diet; vegetarian eating involves adding nutritious alternatives, for example seeds, grains, nuts, pulses, cereals and sprouts. A well-balanced vegetarian diet including all of these and plenty of fresh fruit and vegetables is as nutritious as a well-planned diet containing meat, so even if you do not want to be a full-time vegetarian it is a good idea to have one or two vegetarian days a week. Vegetarians seem to have lower blood pressure and a lower incidence of coronary heart disease than meat eaters.

A vegan diet, containing no meat, milk, eggs, fish or any other animal foods, can be healthy, but regular supplements of vitamin B_{12} are needed as it is found only in animal products.

Eat more fibre

Fibre is the name given to a range of complex carbohydrates found in the cell walls of plants. Also known as roughage, it provides bulk and prevents constipation and intestinal disorders. Fibre

FIBRE CONTENT OF FOOD

High fibre	Medium fibre	Low fibre	No fibre
Bananas	Apples	Boiled potatoes	Butter
Bran	Celery	Cucumber	Cheese
Jacket potatoes	Cornflakes	Grapefruit	Eggs
Brown rice	Green vegetables	Lettuce	Fish
Dried fruits	Muesli	Tomatoes	Meat
Leafy vegetables	Nuts	White bread	Milk
Porridge	Oranges	White rice	Sugar
Pulses			
Rye crispbread			
Sweetcorn			
Wholemeal bread			
Wholewheat pasta			
Rhubarb			

passes through the bowel without being absorbed and it seems to help control levels of cholesterol and sugar in the blood. It also gives you a feeling of satiety without adding too many calories, which is useful if you are trying to lose weight (see page 132).

It is therefore a good idea to make sure that you eat a lot of fibre. Perhaps the simplest way of starting to increase your intake is just to switch from white to wholemeal bread, and then to eat more fibrous foods; the relative fibre values of some foods are given opposite.

FOOD FOR A HEALTHY DIET

Listed below are foods that should be included in your diet, as well as advice on what you can eat in moderation (no more than 3 times per week) and which foods you should avoid. Some foods, such as sugar, chocolate, ice-cream, jam, crisps, cakes, biscuits and pastry, have no nutritional value and should be cut out of your diet.

Meats and other protein foods

Eat as you like: Chicken (skinned); turkey; veal, fish; nuts (except coconut); game such as venison, rabbit and pigeon, egg whites.

Eat in moderation: Lean beef, lamb and pork; eggs.

Avoid: Fatty meats such as spare ribs, liver, brains, kidneys, heart, sweetbreads, sausages, bacon, duck, goose; meat products; salami; smoked fish and shell fish.

Vegetables and fruit

Eat as you like: Broccoli; cabbage; carrots, potatoes cooked in their jackets, sweet potatoes and other root vegetables; spinach and other leafy vegetables; string beans; asparagus; artichokes; sweet corn; tomatoes; strawberries and other berries; fruit such as oranges, grapefruit, melons, tangerines, apricots and peaches; dried fruits; pulses.

Eat in moderation: Potatoes (fried or mashed), yams, broad beans, bananas; avocados.

Breads and cereals

Eat as much as you like: Wholemeal bread, wholegrain rye bread, brown rice, oatmeal, wholewheat pasta, bran.

Eat in moderation: Non-wholewheat pasta, egg noodles, crackers.

Avoid: White bread.

Dairy products

Eat as much as you like: Skimmed milk, cottage cheese, low fat yogurt.

Eat in moderation: Brie, Camembert, Edam, Mozzarella, Ricotta.

Avoid: Full-fat milk, butter, cream, Cheddar, Stilton, cream cheese, Parmesan.

Oils and fats

Eat as much as you like: Polyunsaturated vegetable oils, such as sunflower, corn, safflower, sesame, cotton seed, soya bean.

Eat in moderation: Soft polyunsaturated margarines and monounsaturated oils, such as, olive or groundnut.

Avoid: Lard, suet, butter, vegetable shortening (cocoa butter, palm oil or coconut oil), blended cooking oil, hard margarines.

Drinks

Drink as much as you like: Tea without sugar and herb teas; fruit and vegetable juices; mineral water.

Drink in moderation: Coffee, alcoholic drinks such as wine, fortified wine, beer, cider, spirits.

Avoid: Colas and other carbonated drinks with high sugar content and many artificial additives.

FATS

The consumption of fat in Western countries is very high. For example, in Britain, the average consumption is 100g (4oz) a day. A healthy adult needs no more than 75g (3oz) per day. Therefore consumption should be cut by at least a quarter. However, the problem with fat is not that simple, because it also depends on the type of fat in your diet. There are three main categories of fat found in the diet: saturated, mono-unsaturated and polyunsaturated. The type of fat depends on the number of free links in the chemical structure saturated fats have no free links, mono-unsaturated fats have one, and polyunsaturated fats have more than one.

How do they affect the body?

Saturated fats tend to encourage the liver to produce cholesterol and make the blood more prone to clot. A little cholesterol is needed in the body but less than a quarter of the requirement comes from our food; the remainder is manufactured by the liver. High levels of saturated fats in the diet step up this process, and the excess is deposited on the artery walls in the form of atheroma. Polyunsaturated fats, on the other hand, tend to lower the level of cholesterol in the blood, and they may even reduce the stickiness of the blood platelets. Poly-unsaturated fats therefore play a protective role in helping to keep the walls of the arteries clear. Monounsaturated fats do not increase your cholesterol, but they do not reduce it either.

Not only is our consumption of fat very high – and therefore an important contributory factor to obesity – but more than half of all that fat consumed is saturated. Cutting down on fat generally will not only help to combat weight problems but, better still, a low-fat diet

can stop and may actually reverse existing atherosclerosis. It is particularly important to reduce the amount of saturated fat in your diet and to make sure that what fat you do eat is, as far as possible, polyunsaturated.

Which foods contain fats?

No one food contains only a single type of fat; it is the relative proportion of the different types of fats within a food that makes the food healthy or unhealthy. In general, saturated fats tend to be solid at room temperature and to come from animal sources, whereas polyunsaturated fats are soft, or in the form of oil, and come from vegetables and fish.

Saturated fats are found in beef, lamb, pork and poultry and in all processed meat products such as bacon, sausages, frankfurters and meat pies. Mince bought from a butcher usually has a rather high fat content. You can avoid this source of fat by buying lean meat and mincing it yourself.

Poultry, or white meat, contains less fat than red meat, especially when the skin is removed. Game, such as rabbit, venison, pigeon and pheasant is the leanest meat of all and contains much more polyunsaturated fat and less saturated fat than other meats. Duck and goose are fatty meats but the fat is rather less saturated than red meats.

Milk and most dairy products, such as butter, cheese – particularly hard cheeses such as Cheddar – and cream, are high in saturated fat.

Oils which are low in saturates and high in polyunsaturates include, in descending order of polyunsaturated fat content, safflower, soya bean, sunflower, corn (maize), cotton seed and sesame. Olive oil and groundnut (or peanut) oil contain monounsaturated.

CUTTING DOWN ON FAT

- Eat poultry and game in preference to red meat and meat products. Remove the skin from chicken and other poultry.
- Eat more fish.
- If you do eat red meat, trim away any fat before cooking.
- Grill or bake rather than fry. Cook meat on a rack so that the fat can drain.
- If you do fry, use polyunsaturated oil rather than butter or lard and a non-stick pan so that you use only a very small amount of oil to prevent it sticking.
- Bought mince often contains a lot of fat so it's best to buy lean stewing beef, cut off all visible fat and mince it yourself. Fry mince without adding any fat and then drain off all the fat before you add flavourings.
- Use polyunsaturated margarine instead of butter and spread it sparingly.
- Avoid hard cheeses, such as Cheddar and Stilton, and cream cheese, and buy lower-fat cheeses, such as Edam, Camembert or, even better, cottage or curd cheese as an alternative.
- Change from full-fat milk to semi-skimmed or, best of all, skimmed.
- Use plain low-fat yogurt instead of cream, mayonnaise or salad cream.
- Boil or poach eggs (and no more than three a week) rather than scramble or fry with oil or butter.
- Eat more vegetarian meals or stretch small amounts of meat by mixing them with pulses and vegetables.
- Eat baked or boiled potatoes in preference to chips.
- Avoid manufactured foods, such as biscuits, cakes, pastry, sauces and crisps, that are rich in "hidden" fat, which is usually saturated. If you must eat cakes, make your own using a healthy, polyunsaturated fat.

But beware: just because a food label tells you that a food contains vegetable fat, it does not necessarily mean that it is free from saturated fat; coconut oil, cocoa butter and palm oil (used in commercially prepared biscuits, pie fillings, non-dairy milk and cream substitutes) are all saturated fats. Avoid blended oils because they can be high in saturates.

Even a naturally healthy, polyunsaturated oil can be turned into a harmful, saturated fat if artificially hardened, a process known as hydrogenation. All margarines, for example, contain some hydrogenated fat or they would spill out of the tub, but it's a question of degree; the harder the margarine, the more saturated and the less healthy it is. Margarines which are labelled "high in polyunsaturates" must contain at least 40 per cent of their total fat content as polyunsaturates. Always buy "cold-pressed" oils because they are extracted from the fresh, raw seed; the heat treatment used in some forms of processing can convert some of the polyunsaturated fats into saturated ones.

The advantages of fish

White fish contains hardly any fat at all and is a high-protein, low-fat alternative to meat. Fatty fish, such as mackerel, herring, sardines, tuna, salmon and trout, are excellent sources of polyunsaturated oils.

These oils are believed to have a particularly protective effect on the circulation by making the blood platelets less sticky and consequently less liable to clot. Eskimos, who subsist on large quantities of fish, have a low incidence of heart disease; other research has shown that fish oil supplements can even be helpful to angina patients.

It is a good idea, therefore, to eat fish at least two or three times every week, including fatty fish at least once. And if you eat tinned fish, such as sardines or tuna, choose ones in a named, healthy oil, such as soya or olive.

SUGAR

Despite widespread knowledge that sugar rots your teeth and contributes to obesity, sugar consumption remains high in the Western world. Less than half of the sugar consumed in Britain, for example, is bought as bags of sugar; the rest comes in sweets, cakes, carbonated drinks, fruit squashes and processed foods (including savoury ones).

Sugar is thought by some researchers to contribute to the risk of coronary heart disease, though no one knows for certain why this should be so, the evidence being partly confounded by the fact that those who consume a lot of sugar also tend to consume a lot of fat, which causes its own problems. Sugar tends to cause an increase in the level of blood triglycerides (see pages 45 to 46). There has also been some recent research on the effects of sugar on the rest of the circulation, which suggests that excess sugar is turned, in the liver, into fat – most of which is saturated. The evidence is not, as yet, conclusive.

Cut down on sugar

What is certain is that most of us need to reduce the amount of sugar we eat. This includes not only packet sugar whether white, brown or raw unrefined cane or beet sugar, but also sugar in processed foods, where it may be listed as sugar, sucrose, syrup, dextrose, molasses or caramel. If you must eat sweeteners, use honey or fruit juice concentrates, which contain natural sugars, fructose and glucose, as well as minerals and vitamins.

CUTTING DOWN ON SUGAR

- Drink unsweetened fruit juices, diluted with mineral water if necessary.
- Do not eat sweets.
- Eat fruit at the end of a meal rather than a sticky pudding and munch a piece of fruit as a snack rather than sweets or chocolate.
- Halve the amount of sugar in recipes.
- Read the list of ingredients on processed foods, both sweet and savoury, and do not buy them if they contain sugar.

SODIUM AND POTASSIUM

These are two minerals, which must be present in the correct amounts for the growth and proper functioning of the body. A delicate balance of sodium and potassium is important if the kidneys are to work properly, so that the body can maintain the correct fluid levels.

Salt consumption

An adult needs to eat only 1 gram of salt a day but in many instances we consume far more than is needed. For example, the British eat about 10g (⅓oz) of salt, or sodium chloride, a day. All fruits, vegetables, milk, meats and cereals contain small amounts of sodium. We get

enough from these sources, and the addition of extra salt is unnecessary.

A high consumption of salt is thought by many doctors to be a risk factor in high blood pressure, which is, in turn, a risk factor in coronary heart disease and strokes. Most healthy people can get rid of excess sodium through the kidneys and it does not cause them any harm. However, some people are sensitive to sodium and it is in these people that excessive sodium may cause high blood pressure. If the kidneys fail to eliminate sufficient sodium, or if the heart fails to pump blood efficiently, sodium will accumulate in the body. This excess sodium causes the body to retain water, thus expanding the volume of blood and possibly causing swelling of ankles and other parts of the body.

If you have high blood pressure or a heart or kidney condition, you may be told to reduce the sodium in your diet drastically. If this is impossible or ineffective, the doctor may prescribe a diuretic drug to help the kidneys to get rid of excess fluid and salt (see page 72).

Cutting down on salt does not guarantee a reduction in risks but it certainly will not do you any harm. And even if you don't yet have high blood pressure, it is still a good idea to limit your salt intake before doctor's orders leave you no alternative. The longer you continue to add a lot of salt to your food, the more accustomed you will be to it and the harder it is to cut down.

The problem of hidden salt

About three-quarters of the salt we eat is added to processed foods, which also contain sodium in many other guises: monosodium glutamate (flavour enhancer); sodium bicarbonate (baking powder); sodium cyclamate and sodium saccharin (artificial sweeteners); sodium nitrite, sodium sulphite and sodium benzoate (preservatives). Look out for anything with the word "sodium" or its chemical symbol "Na" in the list of ingredients. Some over-the-counter medicines also contain sodium without it being labelled, so check with your doctor before taking unprescribed medicines. In general, manufacturers should be encouraged to reduce the amount of salt they use. In the meantime, however, if you eat a lot of processed foods, opt for the salt-free or low-salt variety where you have a choice – as in polyunsaturated margarine, breakfast cereals and some tinned vegetables, for example.

CUTTING DOWN ON SALT

■ Start by adding it either during cooking or at the table – never both. Then, as your taste buds adapt, gradually cut salt out of your diet altogether.
■ Use salt substitutes or low-sodium salts or alternative flavourings such as lemon juice, spices or herbs.
■ Avoid highly salted foods such as salami, bacon, ham, sausages, frankfurters, crisps, stock cubes, processed cheese, salted nuts, pickles, olives, ketchup, soy sauce and smoked fish.
■ Keep an eye on your children's eating habits as a taste for over-salted foods is acquired early in life. Never give salt to babies or toddlers whose kidneys are too immature to deal with it.
■ Artificially softened water contains more sodium than hard water, so if you use a domestic water softener, make sure you have a drinking water tap that bypasses it.
■ Read all food and over-the-counter medicine labels carefully for salt content.

Salt added at home accounts for the rest of our salt intake and this is something we can easily control ourselves.

The case for potassium

While our consumption of sodium has increased in recent years, so our consumption of potassium has tended to decrease, because processing removes much of the naturally occurring potassium. Insufficient potassium exaggerates the impact of sodium on the body and it may be this imbalance which produces a rise in blood pressure. There is some evidence that potassium can reduce high blood pressure. Thus it is important not only to reduce the amount of sodium you consume, but also to increase your potassium intake.

Most natural foods contain potassium, and a balanced diet including all the essential foods usually provides sufficient potassium for most people.

Drugs and potassium

Some medications increase the loss of potassium from the kidneys. Diuretics, for example, which are prescribed to rid the body of excess sodium will also eliminate some potassium (see page 73). To counteract this loss, you either have to take a potassium supplement or eat more foods particularly rich in potassium (see below). Some adjustment may also be necessary if you are on a low-sodium diet. Conversely, people with kidney disease may be told to restrict their consumption of potassium.

WHERE TO FIND POTASSIUM

Foods rich in potassium		Foods moderately rich in potassium	
Bananas	Melon	Blackberries	Pears
Beetroot	Nuts	Broccoli	Potatoes (boiled)
Butter beans	Oranges	Brussels sprouts	Spinach
Cabbage	Potatoes (cooked in jacket)	Carrots	Strawberries
Dates		Courgettes	Tomatoes
Figs	Prunes	Milk	Water melon
Grapes	Raisins	Peaches	
Grapefruit (and juice)			

LOSING WEIGHT

One of the benefits of a low-fat, low-sugar, high-fibre way of eating (as outlined in the first part of this chapter) is that you're unlikely to become – or stay – seriously overweight. Limiting your intake of alcohol (see Chapter 11) and regular exercise (see Chapter 14) will also help to keep your weight down.

If you think you need to lose weight, you should first differentiate between just being a little overweight – which is not likely to have much effect on your health – or being downright fat – which can contribute to heart or circulatory disease. To find out where your weight falls, look at the chart opposite.

Not every one puts on weight as a result of eating a lot. Some people have too slow a metabolism, which tends to run in families; others don't take sufficient exercise. Whatever the reason, if you are overweight, your problem is

that you are eating more than you need for your amount of activity.

First of all, drastically reduce your intake of:

● Butter, margarine, cooking fats and oils (avoid fried foods)
● Cheese and cream
● Fatty meat
● Pastries, biscuits and cakes
● Crisps and nuts
● Rich sauces and soups
● Sugary foods including jam, honey, sweets and chocolate
● Alcohol.

Several small meals are better than one (or two) heavy ones, so spread your food throughout the day and do not give in to the temptation of cleaning your plate. Do not allow yourself to get very hungry since you will be tempted to snack on readily available foods like biscuits or sweets. You may find it helpful to arm yourself with a slimming book and to count food calorie values, to join a slimming club, or to ask your doctor's advice, but don't be conned into taking any so-called slimming pills; they do not help in the long run and may actually be harmful to your health.

CUTTING DOWN ON WHAT YOU EAT

Unfortunately, while most diet sheets tell you what to eat and what not to eat, they do not tell you how to resist temptation. Bear in mind that eating is a pleasurable occupation which fulfils not only our nutritional requirements, but also our social and psychological needs.

Parties and eating out

Eating out can present problems. If you are going to a restaurant, tell yourself beforehand that you are going to resist high-calorie food and that you will order only sensible items. Choose fish, but not cooked in a rich sauce, and perhaps a salad (without salad dressing) instead of deep fried vegetables.

At a party, drink mineral water or fruit juice instead of alcohol, or have one drink and sip it slowly to avoid your glass being topped up repeatedly. Allow yourself a limited number of canapes.

At a buffet party it is all too easy to keep piling food on to your plate. To avoid this, walk from one end of the table to the other first, decide what you are going to eat, and only then pick up a plate and serve yourself.

Remember, do not make life impossible by denying yourself everything. You will only go home feeling deprived and annoyed with yourself for refusing

IDEAL WEIGHT CHART

Measure your height without shoes, and weigh yourself without clothes. If you weigh more than the maximum weight for your height and sex, you may be seriously overweight. If you weigh less than the minimum, you should gain some weight.

Height	MEN Acceptable weight	WOMEN Acceptable weight
1.57m (5ft 2in)		46-59kg (102-131lb)
1.60m (5ft 3 in)		48-61kg (105-134lb)
1.63m (5ft 4in)	54-67kg (118-148lb)	49-63kg (108-138lb)
1.65m (5ft 5in)	55-69kg (121-152lb)	50-64kg (111-142lb)
1.68m (5ft 6in)	56-71kg (124-156lb)	52-66kg (114-146lb)
1.70m (5ft 7in)	58-73kg (128-161lb)	54-68kg (118-150lb)
1.73m (5ft 8in)	60-75kg (132-166lb)	55-70kg (122-154lb)
1.75m (5ft 9in)	62-77kg (136-170lb)	57-72kg (126-158lb)
1.78m (5ft 10in)	64-79kg (140-174lb)	59-74kg (130-163lb)
1.80m (5ft 11in)	65-81kg (144-179lb)	61-76kg (134-168lb)
1.83m (6ft)	67-83kg (148-184lb)	63-78kg (138-173lb)
1.85m (6ft 1in)	69-86kg (152-189lb)	
1.88m (6ft 2in)	71-88kg (156-194lb)	
1.90m (6ft 3in)	73-90kg (160-199lb)	

all that delicious food, and probably console yourself with a snack.

Psychological need for food

People sometimes eat in order to satisfy a psychological need. If you eat when your mind is distracted by something else – such as reading or watching television – the food will not satisfy your psychological need and you will be tempted to eat more. To gain the full benefit of eating, switch off the television or put that book down and concentrate on your food.

Food cravings

When you crave for a certain food, do not give in to the impulse straight away. Learning to deny yourself is a necessary part of successful dieting. If the craving persists all day, however, and is still there when you wake up the next morning, it is better to satisfy it with a small amount of the food in question than to let it intensify to the extent that you are in danger of losing control.

One woman in three has cravings for food for three or four days before her period. If you suffer from this problem, either satisfy the cravings with low-calorie snacks or substitute craved-for foods for normal meals.

Diversionary tactics

You may find yourself turning to food for comfort whenever you feel frustrated or angry. Persuade yourself to wait for at least 15 minutes. Once your feelings are under control, you may not feel the need to eat.

If you tend to eat when you feel sorry for yourself or bored, busy yourself with some task that you have been putting off for a long time. You will be surprised how a sense of accomplishment can lift your mood and alleviate the desire to eat.

Keeping the diet going

If you have been successful in losing some weight, it is all too easy to congratulate yourself, or to be influenced by other people's compliments, and to break your diet. Equally do not allow yourself to be discouraged by comments such as "Don't get too skinny, a bit of weight suits you."

The subconscious can sometimes play surprising tricks on your mind. You may, for example, eat something you are not allowed on your diet, then forget all about it. One way of combating this is to keep a food diary and to enter in it everything you eat and drink throughout the day.

The most important thing for you to remember is not to set yourself such over-optimistic, unrealistic goals while you are on your diet. There are bound to be occasions when it simply isn't possible to observe a diet rigorously. Accept that the occasional slip-up is a necessary part of learning a new eating pattern and acquiring new habits.

SELF-HYPNOSIS

Almost any habit can be controlled if you have sufficient motivation. Self-hypnosis is particularly good for helping you to stick to a diet. Try this sequence two or three times a day, preferably before each meal.

Stage one

Sit in a comfortable chair, close your eyes and relax your entire body (see deep muscle relaxation, page 159).

Stage two

When you are completely relaxed, repeat as many of the following phrases to yourself as you are able to remember. Alternatively, pick out one or two that have the most meaning for you and repeat them ten to 20 times each.

● I can see and feel myself as happy and healthy.
● I am in my own private hide-away where I can get to know myself better.
● I see myself entering that hide-away and closing the door.
● I undress and look at my body in my full-length mirror.
● I can see my body clearly.
(Continue for one minute.)

Stage three

Then repeat as many of the following phrases as you can remember:
● Now I can see and feel my body at my ideal weight. (Repeat ten times.)
● My appetite is pleasantly satisfied. (Repeat ten times.)
● I become increasingly comfortable as I attain my desired weight. (Repeat five times.)
● I become healthier and healthier as I attain my desired weight. (Repeat five times.)
● I feel happy and proud of myself as I attain my desired weight. (Repeat five times.)
● I am satisfied with small portions of food. (Repeat five times.)
● I can see and feel my body at my ideal weight and I will carry this image and feeling with me as I return to my normal awareness. (Repeat five times.)
● Now, as I prepare to return to my normal awareness, I bring with me glorious happy feelings. I take a deep breath, open my eyes and stretch comfortably, feeling completely satisfied and full of energy.

ACUPUNCTURE

Some acupuncturists believe that acupuncture can stimulate the brain's satiety centre and thus reduce cravings for food, though its success in this area is more modest than in the area of pain relief. Acupuncture on its own is not likely to be successful unless you have the motivation to lose weight. Most acupuncturists combine acupuncture with other behavioural methods to help a patient stick to a diet.

What will the acupuncturist do?

The most likely treatment is for the acupuncturist to insert needles into your ear at points that are associated with your digestion, tape them in place and leave them there for two to three weeks. If this works, you will notice a change in your appetite and eating habits.

PRINCIPLES OF ACUPUNCTURE

Acupuncture is an ancient Chinese treatment based on the belief that the energy of life, Chi, flows through the body in well defined channels, or meridians. The nature of Chi varies along a continuum, from Yin at one end of the scale to Yang at the other. Yin is dark, cold, solid and female, while Yang is light, warm, hollow and male. The health of the body depends on these two opposing forces being in balance. Any imbalance creates a disharmony, which manifests itself as a disease. Ill-health, then, is regarded as a symptom of an underlying disorder, which will clear up when harmony is restored.

The meridians through which this energy flows form a network over the entire body, but they do not follow the pathways of any system known to Western medicine, corresponding neither to the circulation nor to the nervous system. The heart meridian, for example, runs from the armpit to the tip of the little finger. Acupuncture is a method of stimulating special sensitive points along the meridians using very fine needles, in order to increase or reduce the flow of energy, and thus correct the balance. There is an entire network of meridians on each ear, and some acupuncturists treat patients using only these points. This branch of the therapy is called auricular acupuncture.

11
Alcohol: in moderation

Alcoholic drinks have been enjoyed since the beginning of recorded history. So what's wrong with them?

The short answer, quite simply, is that there is nothing wrong with a very moderate consumption of alcoholic drinks (up to two standard drinks a day, see page 138), even if you have already had a heart attack – that is provided you are used to alcohol, don't start if you are not used to it – but there is plenty wrong with heavy drinking. The difficulty, however, lies in defining exactly what is meant by "heavy". Many of those people who drink more alcohol than is good for their health do so without even realizing how much they're consuming. Put quite simply, the more you drink and the more often you drink, the higher the risk of developing alcohol-related diseases – but because different people can tolerate different levels of alcohol, it is difficult to lay down strict rules.

What is a moderate drinker?
In the main a very moderate drinker is a man who has fewer than 20 drinks in a week or a woman who has less than 13: a heavy drinker is a man who has more than 51 drinks a week or a woman who has more than 36. These definitions may vary slightly from one source to

another, but after reviewing surveys from different parts of the world it becomes obvious that drinking more than two standard drinks per day increases the risk of developing coronary artery disease, high blood pressure and other related diseases, such as peripheral vessel disease or strokes.

Other reasons for limiting intake
There are a great many other compelling reasons for avoiding an excessive consumption of alcohol. Apart from cirrhosis of the liver, excessive drinking can cause brain damage, inflammation of the pancreas and cancer of the digestive tract, mouth, throat and gullet.

Its effect on men and women
Alcohol is absorbed into the blood via the stomach and intestines. It is then quickly and uniformly distributed throughout the body water. Men hold between 55 and 65 per cent of their total body weight in water, in comparison with only 45 to 55 per cent in women. Alcohol is therefore more diluted in men than in women, which is why men can take more alcohol than women. Men are also generally heavier than women of the same size so have more total fluids in their body.

HOW ALCOHOL AFFECTS THE HEART

The precise role of alcohol in heart disease is difficult to assess. There are several reasons for this. The first is the difficulty in establishing links between the two in a particular patient; the only clue may be the patient's self-confessed drinking history. The second reason is that there is evidence to suggest that a small amount of alcohol – not more than the two standard drinks per day – can actually be beneficial to the cardio-vascular system because in these fairly small amounts, alcohol appears to be a relaxant. What is certain, however, is that more than that can contribute to several other risk factors.

Combined with risk factors

For a start, even moderate amounts of alcohol can raise blood pressure in sus-ceptible individuals, while heavy drink-ing can cause, or at least aggravate, high blood pressure. If you are in any doubt about your own susceptibility, consult your doctor. Alcoholics who manage to remain "dry" after withdrawal, have in fact been shown to have lower blood pressure than those who start drinking again. Even small amounts of alcohol can make effective drug treatment very difficult because alcohol can interfere with the medication either by inhibiting the action of the drug or by causing a dangerous reaction

Excess alcohol is thought to raise the levels of cholesterol and triglycerides in the blood and thus to accelerate the process of atherosclerosis (see page 62). Alcohol also gives rise to another harm-ful process known as "coronary steal". Alcohol can cause normal blood vessels to dilate, allowing more blood to flow through them. Blood is correspondingly "stolen" from those arteries which have been narrowed by disease.

People who drink a lot of alcohol are often overweight. As well as being very high in calories – there are 180 calories in the average 600ml (1 pint) of beer – and poor in essential nutrients, alcohol tends to stimulate the appetite. It takes only some simple arithmetic to add the calorific value of everything you drink to that of everything you eat, and it's not difficult to see where a beer gut comes from! Heavy drinkers also tend to take too little exercise, which not only adds to any weight problems but also means that they miss out on all the cardio-vascular benefits that regular physical exercise can bring (see Chapter 14).

Drinking to excess goes hand in hand with several other risk factors. For in-stance, the person who drinks to excess often smokes (see Chapter 12), drinks a lot of coffee (see page 47) and displays Type A behaviour patterns (see page 54). Also, alcohol is closely related to stress, whether as a cause or a symptom.

In view of all these factors, it is hardly surprising that a high consumption of alcohol doubles the risk of suffering a stroke, or that it is extremely common in heart attack victims.

Alcohol after a heart attack

There is no reason for total abstinence, even after a heart attack. In fact, a small amount of alcohol – say, a small glass of sherry or whisky before dinner and a glass of wine with your meal – may help your convalescence by boosting morale, if you are used to drinking. Total pro-hibition could cause a great deal of stress, which could well be more harm-ful than a modest quantity of alcohol.

Alcohol is, however, a mild depress-ent of the heart muscle and it can, in excessive amounts, lead to further trouble in those people whose hearts are particularly sensitive to it. It can weaken the heart's pumping ability or bring on rhythm irregularities which manifest themselves as palpitations. If these occur, it is best to abstain, and anyone whose heart attack has resulted in heart failure should abstain. Indeed, whatever form of heart disease you suffer from, you should be especially temperate in your approach to alcohol.

WHAT IS MODERATION?

The key to the whole subject of alcohol is moderation, but what exactly is that? Obviously not all alcoholic drinks are the same: what counts is how much pure alcohol they contain. This varies from country to country, but is about

HOW DIFFERENT DRINKS COMPARE

The alcohol content varies tremendously and you must take this into account when estimating your consumption. The following chart should help you calculate your intake.

			Equivalent of "standard" drink
BEERS AND LAGERS	Ordinary strength beer or lager	300ml (½ pint)	1
		600ml (1 pint)	2
		440ml can (¾ pint)	1½
	Strong ale or lager	300ml (½ pint)	2
		600ml (1 pint)	4
		440ml can (¾ pint)	3
	Extra strength beer or lager	300ml (½ pint)	2½
		600ml (1 pint)	5
		440ml can (¾ pint)	4
CIDERS	Ordinary strength cider	300ml (½ pint)	1½
		600ml (1 pint)	3
	Strong cider	300ml (½ pint)	2
		600ml (1 pint)	4
SPIRITS	(whisky, gin, vodka, bacardi, brandy)	1 standard single measure 24-35ml (⅙-¼ gill)	1-1½
		1 bottle	30
WINES	Table wine	1 glass	1
		1 bottle (70cl)	7
		1 litre bottle	10
	Sherry or vermouth	1 standard measure	1
		1 bottle	12

three to six per cent in beers and lagers; eight to 14 per cent in table wines; 15 to 20 per cent in sherry; and 30 to 40 per cent in most distilled spirits.

To put it another way, all of the following alcoholic drinks, in bar measures, contain the same amount of alcohol and can be regarded as one "standard" drink.

- 300ml (½ pint) beer or lager
- 30 ml (1 floz) measure of spirits
- 120ml (4 floz) glass of wine
- Measure of sherry or vermouth.

It is important that you are aware that home measures are usually much more generous; one drink at home may, in fact, be equivalent to two, three, or even four "standard" drinks.

What kind of drinker are you?

Calculate how much alcohol you drink by writing down *exactly* what you drank in the last seven days. Also write down when, where and with whom you drank in each case: this will enable you to identify any high-risk times or circumstances if you discover that your consumption is higher than it should be and you need to cut down. Then, using the chart on the opposite page, add up your score. Don't cheat and don't make an excuse that last week was not a typical week.

HOW TO REDUCE YOUR INTAKE

If after working out your weekly total (see above) you find that you habitually drink more than three drinks a day, more than five times a week, you would benefit – not only physically but also socially and financially – by cutting down your consumption. If you decide to reduce your alcohol intake, you may find the following guidelines helpful.

Look at your reasons for drinking

Before you tackle the actual problem of cutting down, look carefully at your weekly drinking chart. See if you can pinpoint those high-risk occasions and circumstances. For example, ask yourself the following questions.

- Do you drink more heavily in certain places – say, a particular wine bar or at home when you're by yourself and feeling lonely?
- Do you drink more with one particular friend or "drinking partner"?
- What is your emotional state when you drink to excess? Is it one of anger, tension, pressure, frustration, depression or happiness?

In fact it is a good idea to keep a record of your drinking habits over a slightly longer period – say two or three weeks – because it may give you a clearer picture of your drinking pattern.

How to revise your drinking habits

Having established the high-risk areas, the first thing to do is to avoid situations in which you are most likely to drink to excess. Try to rearrange your life a little, at least to begin with. Leave work earlier or later so you can avoid your usual time for a drink after work; avoid the company of the person with whom you usually binge; and when you do go for a drink with friends, order a completely different, less alcoholic drink from your usual one.

If you are going out with friends, set yourself a target number of drinks before you start drinking and stick to that limit. Keep a discreet but careful count of your drinks: write it down on a scrap of paper or in your diary, alternatively, make notches on a beermat with your thumbnail, or transfer coins from one pocket to another. Pace your drinking throughout the evening. Sip your drink so that it lasts longer. And if you manage to keep to the limit you set yourself, reward yourself with a special treat – a visit to the theatre, some new clothes, or perhaps an extra hour in bed at the weekend.

The habit of buying rounds is a dangerous one, so if you and your drinking companions regularly buy rounds for one another, it is high time to change that pattern, and to buy your own drinks. Do not worry about this being an unpopular move with your friends: they may even be relieved because buying rounds can be very expensive. Limit yourself to smaller measures than usual – 300ml (½ pints) of beer instead of 600ml (1 pint), single whiskies instead of doubles – or try alternating alcoholic drinks with non-alcoholic ones. If you think that you are likely to drink more than you would like, you might prefer to avoid the event altogether, arrive deliberately late or leave early.

What to tell your friends

If you feel too embarrassed to tell your friends that you're cutting down on your drinking, find some acceptable way of explaining your new-found temperance.
● "I'm trying to save money."
● "Doctor's orders."
● "I'm trying to lose weight."
● "I'm driving."
● "I had too much to drink yesterday/at lunchtime."
● "I'm going out to dinner later."
● "I'm going to the gym."

Above all, remember that getting drunk doesn't make you tall, virile, witty or seductive. These are all advertising ploys to persuade you to spend more money. Calculate how much you could save every year by having just one, or two, or three . . . fewer drinks a day and see what that will buy you.

Relaxed persuasion

Try the following exercise whenever you feel like a drink, or at least two or three times a day. Sit quietly for five minutes and relax all your muscles deeply and in turn (see pages 159 to 162). When you are feeling completely relaxed, repeat one or two of the following phrases to yourself between 15 and 20 times, either silently or aloud.
● "I am becoming freer and freer from alcohol and feeling happier and happier every day."
● "As each day goes by, I am able to abstain from alcohol for longer and longer periods."
● "I am in perfect control of my drinking and I am proud of this."
● "I foresee myself as happy and free from alcohol."
● "I am calm and relaxed and free from alcohol."

As you prepare to return to your normal awareness, imagine feeling full of health and happiness. Take a deep breath and open your eyes slowly, feeling peaceful and serene. Stretch your body, and as you do so you will feel refreshed and full of energy.

HEAVY DRINKERS

If you are a heavy drinker, never stop drinking suddenly. If your body has become accustomed to a certain regular intake of alcohol, you may suffer severe withdrawal symptoms if you try to go "cold turkey". One of these symptoms is a feeling of chilliness, combined with goose pimply skin (it is this similarity to the skin of a plucked turkey that gave rise to the term "cold turkey"). Another far more debilitating symptom of withdrawal is delirium tremens, or DTs, which is characterized by feelings of confusion, anxiety, paranoia, delusion, hallucination and possible fits.

Aim at first to reach a moderate level of drinking (i.e., a maximum of 36 standard drinks per week for men, 24 per week for women) by gradually cutting down your overall level by five drinks each week. If your present level is 51 or more drinks a week (36 or more for women), cut down by ten a week until you reach 50 (35 for women), and then by five a week until you reach the moderate level. If you have high blood pressure, have had a heart attack, or your doctor has told you that your heart is particularly sensitive to alcohol, you will have to continue until you are having no more than two drinks per day, or give up altogether.

GETTING OUTSIDE HELP

Cutting down gradually is much easier if you have the support of your family and friends. If you live on your own, or if you have had trouble cutting down, you might benefit from some outside help. Talk to your doctor who, depending on the extent of your problem, may refer you to one of the many centres that help people come off, and stay off, alcohol. In some instances, a course of acupuncture (see page 135) or hypnotherapy may help. Ask your doctor if he can recommend anyone. You should try to make sure you find a therapist with experience in this area (see Useful addresses, page 187).

Hospital admission

If you are a heavy drinker and you have tried to give up or cut down several times, you need medication for high blood pressure or are suffering from any condition that requires you not to drink alcohol, your doctor may arrange for you to be admitted to hospital for "drying out". If this does happen, you will probably be treated as follows. During the first day you will be given six drinks, a large dose of tranquillizer and an anti-convulsive drug to prevent you having fits. The number of drinks you are allowed will be reduced by one each day and the amount of tranquillizers and anti-convulsive drugs will be reduced in proportion. You will probably stay in hospital for anything between ten days and four weeks. Before you are discharged from hospital, you will be put in touch with your local branch of Alcoholics Anonymous or a similar organization. These organizations have a 24 hour telephone number which you can use any time you need advice or support. They also organize regular meetings where you can discuss your problem with professional counsellors or other people in the same position as yourself. See Useful addresses, page 187, for other organizations that can help you.

HELPING SOMEONE CUT DOWN

Everyone should respect the aims and wishes of the person who wants to drink in moderation, to cut down, or even to abstain completely. The following guidelines may help you to help anyone who is trying to avoid excessive alcohol:

■ Never insist on topping up someone's glass if they do not want you to.

■ Don't insist on including someone in a round of drinks if they would prefer to buy their own drink.

■ Always provide non-alcoholic drinks if you are entertaining.

■ Always provide something to eat with alcoholic drinks, as food delays the absorption of alcohol into the body.

■ Recognize your responsibility in preventing drunken driving and make sure that any guests who are driving home do not leave your house drunk. This does not mean plying them with coffee before they leave: it means they should either drink or drive, not both.

12
Smoking: giving up

If you really want to give up smoking, you will. The key to success is strong motivation; and the key to strong motivation is to be fully informed.

Recent medical research has proved, beyond doubt, that smoking is a dangerous habit. The British Medical Research Council's working party investigating the treatment of mild hypertension has recently published the results of its study in which some 18,000 men and women took part. The patients were divided into two groups, with smokers and non-smokers in each group. One group was treated with drugs, while the other group was given placebo, or dummy tablets. The results showed that, after five years, there was very little difference between the two groups in terms of heart attacks and strokes, though a considerable number of those taking drugs suffered unpleasant side-effects. There was, however, a significant difference between smokers and non-smokers, and those who did not smoke fared much better. In other words, the advantages of not smoking far outweighed the questionable benefits of swallowing pills for several years to try to control mild high blood pressure.

Smoking and the link with coronary heart disease
Smoking causes more deaths from coronary heart disease – the single biggest killer of the Western world – than from any other smoking-related disease. The risk of having a heart attack rises with the number of cigarettes smoked but, in general, people who smoke are twice as likely to die from a heart attack as those who do not smoke. The younger you are when you start smoking, the greater the relative risk.

Smoking and other diseases
There are, of course, a large number of other diseases which are either directly caused by, or aggravated by, smoking, including strokes, chronic bronchitis, emphysema, respiratory failure and lung cancer. Smoking is also closely associated with peripheral vessel disease (see page 26) which can, in the most severe cases, result in gangrene and amputation of the affected leg. Over 95 per cent of those suffering from this disease are cigarette smokers.

If you already have heart disease
Smoking is particularly dangerous if you have already suffered a heart attack or if you are subject to bouts of angina. Indeed, the risk of having a fatal heart attack is markedly increased if you continue to smoke, in spite of such clear-cut warnings. If you stop smoking after a heart attack, you stand about half the chance of another attack. This "treatment" has a better record than either drugs or surgery and, best of all, it is something you can do for yourself.

HOW SMOKING AFFECTS THE HEART

Tobacco smoke is a complex mixture of some 4,000 chemicals, the most significant of which are nicotine and carbon monoxide. Nicotine stimulates the production of stress hormones such as noradrenaline and adrenaline. These hormones make the heart beat harder and faster, causing a temporary rise in blood pressure as well as increasing the heart's oxygen demand. Healthy coronary arteries can dilate to increase the supply of blood to the heart, but if the arteries are affected by atherosclerosis, they are not able to meet the increased demand.

Carbon monoxide is an odourless, but poisonous gas which combines with haemoglobin in the blood, in competition with oxygen, and thus causes a relative oxygen deficiency. Both nicotine and carbon monoxide can cause the blood platelets to become sticky and clot more readily, thus increasing the risk of thrombosis. These clots in the bloodstream can damage the delicate lining of the arteries and hasten the development of atherosclerosis (see page 63).

Inhalation allows large amounts of nicotine and carbon monoxide to enter the bloodstream. Cigarettes are therefore much more closely associated with the risk of heart disease than pipes or cigars, because pipe and cigar smokers do not usually inhale. However, cigarette smokers who switch to a pipe or cigars often continue to inhale and, as a result, may not reduce their risk by making the switch. Similarly, smokers who change to low-tar brands tend to inhale more deeply in order to maintain their nicotine intake.

YOUR QUESTIONS ANSWERED

One of the reasons that so many people continue to smoke is their ability to develop a particular kind of logic which they use to justify their habit. The following are some of the arguments they resort to. See if you can identify yourself. If you can, I hope that the counter-argument will convince you to stop.

● *Uncle John smoked a packet a day and lived to be a hundred.*
Some people live to a great age despite their efforts to the contrary. They are the exceptions that prove the rule. It does not mean that they live healthy lives.

● *It is too hard to stop. I just don't have the willpower.*
No one would claim that giving up smoking is easy: it isn't, but it isn't impossible. There are some 11 million ex-smokers in the UK, and 35 million in the USA to prove it.

● *If I stop smoking, I will put on weight. Isn't that just as dangerous?*
It is true that non-smokers have a better appetite and digestion than smokers, and also that people who have recently stopped smoking tend to nibble more between meals. However, if you are careful and watch your calories, you will not put on weight. But even if you do, smoking is incomparably more dangerous than putting on weight.

● *Smoking helps me to concentrate.*
Yes, after a cigarette, smokers tend to feel sharper for a while because nicotine mobilizes the release of adrenaline and noradrenaline into the bloodstream (see above). But this is only a temporary phenomenon: once the effect wears off, you feel worse and you need another cigarette, then another . . . hence the vicious trap of addiction.

● *Smoking helps me to relax.*
A lot of people say that, even though physiologically it is not true. Cigarettes are actually a stimulant. They speed up the action of your heart (see page 143). The real reason people find smoking relaxing is that it is a good excuse to take a break from whatever they are doing.

● *I've smoked for so many years now, isn't it too late to stop?*
No, it isn't. The risk of becoming ill, as well as of dying from some smoking-related disease, falls steadily in everyone who gives up smoking, regardless of their age. The risk decreases particularly quickly within the first year of giving up, and after five to ten years it approaches that of someone who has never smoked.

● *But I don't smoke as much as I used to. I only smoke 15 cigarettes a day now compared with the 50 or 60 I used to smoke.*
Well done! If you can reduce your intake that much you are capable of stopping. So why don't you give up altogether? You will lose your smoker's cough, your breathing will improve, you will feel much fitter, your food will taste better – and so will you!

● *I don't really inhale so it can't be very bad for my health.*
It is true that inhaling increases the dangers of smoking, but some nicotine is absorbed even if you don't inhale.

● *I have tried to give up hundreds of times, but I just can't seem to stick at it.*
This is true of lots of people. Most ex-smokers try several times before they succeed. You can only succeed by persevering. Maybe you have now learnt enough about your particular problem to succeed next time.

● *I become so irritable when I try to stop smoking that my partner tells me to start smoking again.*
Although it can be a difficult time, no one has ever died of temporary irritability, which is more than can be said of smoking! Keep at it, and this difficult patch will last only a little while.

● *At least I'm not harming others, so why don't people stop preaching and leave us smokers alone?*
You are wrong. There is now evidence to suggest that the non-smoker who passively and involuntarily inhales "sidestream" smoke (from the end of the cigarette) in fact takes in a much higher concentration of noxious substances than the smoker who actually inhales "mainstream" smoke. Passive smoking may be particularly harmful to those who suffer from heart disease or angina.

The spouse and children of a smoker also have a higher incidence of chest infections and cancers and, on average, die four years earlier than those who are not exposed to cigarette fumes.

WHY DO YOU SMOKE?

Having read through all of the above questions you should now be aware that giving up smoking is essential because it will improve the quality of your life as well as that of anyone around you – your partner, children or colleagues. However, before you can give up smoking, it is important that you understand what kind of smoker you are, and why and when you smoke. The questionnaire opposite may help you find out. Turn to page 146 to analyze your score.

Analyzing your reasons
Complete the questionnaire on the opposite page and add up your score. Scores can vary from 3 to 15. Any score of 11 and above is high; any score of 7

WHAT KIND OF SMOKER ARE YOU?

How often do your feelings about smoking coincide with the following statements? Circle the number in each case which best applies to you.

Statement	Always	Often	Occasionally	Rarely	Never
A I smoke cigarettes in order to keep myself going	5	4	3	2	1
B Handling a cigarette is part of the enjoyment of smoking it	5	4	3	2	1
C Smoking cigarettes is pleasant and relaxing	5	4	3	2	1
D I light up a cigarette when I feel angry about something	5	4	3	2	1
E When I have run out of cigarettes, I find it almost unbearable until I can get some more	5	4	3	2	1
F I smoke cigarettes automatically, without even being aware of it	5	4	3	2	1
G I smoke cigarettes to stimulate me, to perk myself up	5	4	3	2	1
H Part of the enjoyment of smoking a cigarette comes from the steps I take to light up	5	4	3	2	1
I I find cigarettes pleasurable	5	4	3	2	1
J When I feel uncomfortable or upset about something I light up a cigarette	5	4	3	2	1
K I am very much aware that I miss cigarettes when I am not smoking	5	4	3	2	1
L I light up a cigarette without realizing I still have one burning in the ashtray	5	4	3	2	1
M I smoke cigarettes to give me a "lift"	5	4	3	2	1
N When I smoke a cigarette, part of the enjoyment is watching the smoke as I exhale it	5	4	3	2	1
O I most want a cigarette when I am comfortable and relaxed	5	4	3	2	1
P I smoke when I feel "blue" or want to take my mind off my worries	5	4	3	2	1
Q I get a real gnawing hunger for a cigarette when I haven't smoked for a while	5	4	3	2	1
R I've found a cigarette in my mouth and didn't remember putting it there	5	4	3	2	1

How to score

Enter the numbers you have circled for each of the questions in the spaces below, putting the number you have circled after Question A over the letter A, after Question B over the letter B, and so on. Now add up the three scores within each category. For example, the sum of your scores over A, G and M, gives you your score for Stimulation, B, H and N your score of Handling and so on. Turn to page 146 to analyze the score.

	Total					Total	
__ + __ + __ =	Stimulation			__ + __ + __ =	"Crutch": tension relief		
A G M			D	J	P		
__ + __ + __ =	Handling			__ + __ + __ =	"Craving": psychological addiction		
B H N			E	K	Q		
__ + __ + __ =	Relaxation			__ + __ + __ =	Habit		
C I O			F	L	R		

and below is low. A score of 11 or more indicates a particular source of satisfaction in that category. You will either have to learn to do without that specific area of satisfaction, or find some other more acceptable means of satisfying it. Here are some of my suggestions.

Stimulation

If your score is high in this area, it is likely that cigarettes help you to wake up, stay alert and keep going. So try a brisk walk, a swim, skipping, cycling or jogging to redirect your energies.

Handling

Handling things can be satisfying but you can keep your hands busy without lighting up a cigarette. Try toying with a pencil or some worry beads. My father used to keep a watch in his waistcoat pocket secured by a long, gold chain to one of the buttons; whenever he had a problem he used to roll this chain between his fingers. And if you must also put something in your mouth, try chewing gum or sucking a mint.

Relaxation

A number of people say that they smoke because they enjoy the sensation of relaxation it brings. In fact, they smoke to prevent themselves from feeling bad. If you have a high score in this area, try substituting other pleasurable activities

like eating, drinking and social activities which, within limits, are harmless. Better still, learn a relaxation routine to ease tension (see pages 158 to 167).

"Crutch": tension relief

Some smokers use cigarettes as "tranquillizers" in moments of stress or discomfort, learn one of the relaxation techniques on pages 158 to 167, rather than relying on a cigarette.

"Craving": psychological addiction

If you smoke because you are addicted to nicotine, you will begin to crave for the next cigarette the minute you put one out. When you give up, it will be easier to do so abruptly and completely or try aversion therapy (see page 149). Alternatively, you could try nicotine gum (see page 149).

Habit

If you smoke out of sheer habit, you can't be getting much satisfaction out of it. You may find it surprisingly easy to stop if you can disrupt the habit pattern that has built up around the act of smoking. Change to another brand, keep cigarettes and lighter or matches in different places. Learn to ask yourself, "Do I really want this cigarette?" every time you reach for one. You will be amazed at how often the answer is no.

GIVING UP

Some people do find it easy to give up smoking and stick to it. Others, however, do not. I have outlined a few ways that may help. These include deciding on a date in advance and either giving up abruptly and completely (the "cold turkey" approach) or gradually over a period of two or three weeks. There's no

doubt that the "cold turkey" approach works best for most people.

If you are finding it particularly difficult, remember that your doctor may be able to help you. Doctors are, for obvious reasons, particularly keen to encourage people to give up this dangerous habit and your doctor may, for example, be able to recommend an anti-smoking clinic or group, or prescribe nicotine gum (see page 149).

A LONG-TERM STRATEGY

If you find it very difficult to give up smoking, try following this long-term plan of action.

Stage one

Decide on the date and time at which you will stop smoking. About two or three weeks ahead is sufficient time in which to prepare yourself but choose your date carefully. It might be foolish to attempt to give up just before Christmas, for example, when you will have a lot of social pressures. Many people find it easiest to choose the end of a particular project at work, a long weekend or a holiday, when they're not under too much stress. Formalize your resolution in writing and get a friend to witness your signature.

Stage two

Next monitor your smoking pattern. Planning the best strategy to stop smoking, and learning to cope with the discomfort it entails before your actual target day arrives, will improve your chances of success. In order to plan the right strategy, you need to understand your smoking pattern.

One of the best ways of doing this is to make a note each time you smoke a cigarette, recording time and place, what you are doing and how important that particular cigarette is to you on a 1-5 scale. If you want that cigarette very badly, score 1; if it is unimportant, score 5; and so on – a sample record is given below. Wrap your record sheet round your packet of cigarettes; continue to keep it until your target date.

After several days of self-monitoring, look at your smoking pattern and identify those situations which give rise to the strongest desire to smoke. Once you have identified the "high risk" situations, you can lay the groundwork for combating them.

Stage three

Enlist the support of other people. Giving up smoking can be both difficult and lonely and, as a result, a lot of people feel an increased sense of irritability and anxiety. It will help if you can find a friend or relative who will encourage and support you. Explain that you may well need to contact him frequently and that he can help you by acknowledging your problem and by reinforcing your expectation of success. Plan plenty of non-smoking activities together that will keep you busy during times of "high risk".

SAMPLE SMOKING RECORD

Day/Date	Time	Place	Activity while smoking	Value rating 1-5*
Monday 16/7	7.00 a.m.	Bedroom	Just getting up	4
Monday 16/7	8.40 a.m.	Car	Driving	2
Monday 16/7	10.30 a.m.	At work	Having coffee	1
Monday 16/7	12.10 p.m.	At work	On the telephone	2

*Value rating 1 = most important 5 = least important

USEFUL TIPS

- Throw away all your cigarettes so there are none around to tempt you, and throw away all your smoking paraphernalia, including your lighter, matches, cigarette holder, and ashtrays.
- Most smokers feel like smoking immediately after a meal, so don't sit around; leave the table immediately and start something else.
- Whenever you experience an urge to smoke, take between five and ten deep breaths and relax.
- Go to the dentist when you give up and have your teeth cleaned and polished.
- Avoid coffee, alcohol and any other beverage which you normally associate with smoking. Change to herb tea, fruit juice or mineral water instead. It is particularly important to avoid any heavy drinking, not simply because it is in itself very bad for your health (see Chapter 11), but also because alcohol can play havoc with people's resolve.
- Give up at the same time as someone else who smokes and contact each other daily for encouragement.
- Let other people know that you have given up and ask them not to offer you cigarettes, and if possible, not to smoke while you are in the same room.
- Write down all the positive things about yourself you have noticed since you stopped smoking, such as fresher breath, easier breathing, more stamina, cleaner teeth, healthier gums, a better sense of smell and taste, and fresher-smelling clothes and hair, not to mention a feeling of tremendous achievement.
- Write down all your reasons for wanting to give up and refer to your list from time to time, to remind yourself how important it is to give up.
- Whenever you want a cigarette, chew gum, suck a peppermint or nibble a raw carrot instead.
- Put aside the money you're saving from not smoking and use it to buy yourself a treat, perhaps to celebrate your first (and subsequent) cigarette-free anniversary.

GIVING UP IN STAGES

Some people can give up only if they cut down gradually. If you are sure that this method will suit you better, observe the following useful rules. In general, start gradually increasing the length of time between cigarettes during the first week. Increase the interval between cigarettes to at least two hours during the second week. Then go on widening the gap and finally, give up altogether.

● **Do not smoke in bed** Resolve to keep your bedroom fresh so that you can at least breathe smoke-free air all night. You can gradually ban smoking in other places, such as the bathroom, the car, or not in front of the children.

● **Do not smoke first thing in the morning** Start the day right. Once you have had your first cigarette, you will have another, and another. The longer you can put off the first one, the easier it will be to go without.

● **Do not smoke before breakfast** Smoking before breakfast irritates the lining of your stomach and you're more likely to develop a peptic ulcer.

● **Do not smoke while travelling** Sit in the no-smoking area of the bus, train or aeroplane.

● **Do not smoke less than an hour before a meal** Smoking suppresses your appetite and ruins your sense of smell and taste. Yet the whole enjoyment of the meal lies in its aroma and flavour. Why spoil it?

● **Do not smoke the whole cigarette** Smoke progressively less of each cigarette before stubbing it out, and reduce the depth of your inhalation.

● **Do not smoke during a meal** You probably eat with other people. Have some consideration and don't spoil their enjoyment as well as your own.

● **Smoke only one cigarette after a meal** Most smokers find that the cigarette they light up immediately after a meal is the most enjoyable one of all and, hence, it is the most difficult one to give up. Tackle that cigarette last of all but, meanwhile, make sure that you smoke only the one.

● **Do not smoke more than one cigarette every hour** If you can persuade yourself that you can have a cigarette in just a few more minutes, you won't feel too desperate. Make the interval a little longer each day.

● **Do not smoke less than an hour before going to bed** This cigarette is possibly the least important one in the day for you anyway, because by this time your throat is dry and your mouth parched as a result of all the others you've consumed. It is also likely to be the most harmful because of the high concentration of tar in your lungs throughout the night.

AVERSION THERAPY

There are ways in which you can condition yourself against smoking by teaming cigarettes with noxious stimuli. These give cigarettes unpleasant associations and put you off smoking. They can include sitting in a hot, stuffy, smoky atmosphere, eating tablets that make cigarettes taste revolting or locking yourself in a small room and chain smoking until you feel so dizzy and sick that you never want to smoke again.

HYPNOSIS

Some people find hypnosis of great value. It's a simple procedure, whereby the therapist suggests to you the benefits of not smoking while you are in a highly suggestible hypnotic trance. The important thing about it is that, for it to work, you must want to give up.

Alternatively, you can try using self-hypnosis. Relax deeply (see page 158) and then repeat, about 15 to 20 times, phrases such as:

● "Smoking doesn't matter, I can breathe better in fresh air."
● "I am becoming freer and freer from nicotine and feeling happier and happier."
● "I am in perfect control of my health and I am proud of my accomplishment."
● "I am calm and relaxed and free from cigarettes."

NICOTINE CHEWING GUM

Chewing gum containing nicotine, or Nicorette, is available on prescription. There are two ways in which it can help:
● It provides a substitute oral activity.
● It relieves withdrawal symptoms caused by nicotine dependence.

How do you take it?

Nicotine gum comes in two strengths, 2mg and 4mg. You simply break off a small piece and chew it like chewing gum. Nicotine is slowly released and absorbed through the surface of the mouth. Follow the instructions on the packet carefully. If you are sufficiently motivated to stop, it can help, but don't smoke and chew the gum as this would merely step up your nicotine intake.

ACUPUNCTURE

Some smokers find acupuncture (see page 135) helps them give up, but it still requires strong motivation to succeed. It is more effective in those who smoke 20 or more cigarettes a day.

The ear is first cleansed with surgical spirit. A sterile acupuncture needle is then inserted into the area of each ear which corresponds to the lungs and taped in place. Some people are asked not to disturb the needle, others are told to pull the lobe of the ear every time they have a keen desire to smoke. The needle will be left in place for two weeks unless any infection develops.

13
Coping with stress

When stress becomes so excessive or prolonged that it becomes a way of life, it can contribute, in a susceptible individual, to the development of high blood pressure or coronary heart disease (see pages 49 to 61).

The sources of stress are numerous, but the way in which the body reacts to them is always the same. The degree to which the stress response is mobilized differs from person to person, but the basic mechanism does not change (see pages 51 to 52). In order to reduce stress in your life, you have to either remove the sources of stress or change your habitual response: the latter is far easier than trying to change the rest of the world to fit in with you!

Various different systems of stress management have been evolved, all of which necessitate developing an insight into your own problems and personality, and then taking the responsibility for dealing with those problems. For some people, it is necessary only to learn a simple relaxation technique and to spend a few minutes daily practising it. Others may need to seek professional advice, or to concentrate on spiritual matters and on finding a meaning to life beyond that of mundane, day-to-day living and materialistic goals.

STRESS MANAGEMENT

The things I have found most useful in helping my patients to reduce stress in their lives are listed below. I call them the ten "A" commandments: Awareness, Avoidance, Anticipation, Action, Appraisal, Amnesty, Assertiveness, Anger management, Altering your perspectives, Assisted relaxation.

AWARENESS
Your first task is to understand what stress is and how it can put undue strain on your health. You also need to be able to recognize its onset and its biological or behavioural symptoms. This awareness is in itself very important because unless and until you know exactly what is wrong, you cannot begin to reduce the impact of stress on your life.

You may, for example, be vaguely aware that you sometimes display signs of stress without understanding exactly why this should be so, because you do not take a mental note of stressful situations. The next time you feel you are under stress, think about what produced it, how you reacted, what you said, and how you felt.

Here is an example:
● *What was the situation?*
A car cut in sharply in front of me. I was worried about being late.

● *What was your reaction?*
Anger at the driver of that car.
● *What did you say?*
Stupid man! Who does he think he is?
● *How did you feel afterwards?*
Tense, slight palpitations. It took me some time to get back to my thoughts about the lecture I was due to give a few minutes later.

We all know that such things as someone cutting in suddenly, or a particularly slow driver in front of you, are inevitable occurrences on the road, yet they give rise all too easily to the body's primitive responses such as the "fight or flight" reflex (see page 51).

Once you are aware of your stress responses, you need to remind yourself that there is no need to react every time as if it were a question of life and death. Decide how you will react and what you will say in future when confronted with similar situations.

AVOIDANCE

You do not have to try to avoid stress altogether, even if you could. A certain amount provides a creative challenge and zest for life provided you know when to withdraw; overloading your capacities can only be harmful. You must learn to recognize your limits, be prepared to accept them, and then avoid exposing yourself to the most explosive situations or continuing to the point of exhaustion. The key word, as in all things, is balance.

ANTICIPATION

If stress is unavoidable, you should at least learn to anticipate it, be prepared for it and thus reduce its harmful impact on your health. If you can't avoid it, you might as well acknowledge it. The bills will not go away if you don't open your mail; you can expect a legal summons if you don't pay your parking fines; and a relationship can only become sour if you do not attempt to smooth out conflicts straight away. So anticipate problems before they occur and do everything you can to reduce their impact.

ACTION

If you can neither avoid stress nor anticipate it, you should at least try to channel the energy which is unleashed by the stress response in a more creative way. As I explained in Chapter 5, unless this energy is dissipated, it can hit back at you and provoke various disorders of the body. So how do you channel this energy more positively? When you feel angry, for example, telephone a friend and get it off your chest or, as an alternative, walk it off. If you feel frustrated by bureaucracy or by the inflexible attitudes of your colleagues at work, burn off this energy by playing a game of tennis, or going for a swim. Gentle rhythmic exercise, like swimming, cycling and walking, is a superb way of relaxing mind and body, and releasing tensions caused by the stresses of everyday life. Regular exercise also ensures a good night's sleep, after which you wake up refreshed. Exercise is discussed in more detail in Chapter 14.

APPRAISAL

Some people go to pieces because they imagine a certain situation to be far more intimidating than it really is. Now that you know the purpose of the "fight or flight" response (see page 51), ask yourself if your stress response is really appropriate to the situation every time you feel angry or stressed. There is evidence from some studies that those people who refuse to recognize stress, or redefine a previously stressful situation, seem to become less anxious about it and to suffer a less intense, less protracted physiological response.

AMNESTY

Long-standing grudges, hatred and resentments, whether rooted in real or imaginary events, can generate a great deal of stress. It is possible, however, to forgive and forget and to wipe the slate clean. If you decide to do that, it is of course much more helpful if you let the other party know. People occasionally ask, "Why open old wounds again and become even more unhappy?" But the fact is that the wound, though old, is still very much alive since it continues to bother you.

ASSERTIVENESS

You may sometimes find it difficult to assert or express your feelings and your desires. Some people tend to bottle up their emotions for fear of causing any unpleasantness or arguments. Suppressing emotions can lead to frustration and to low self-esteem. Being assertive, on the other hand, means that you are able to stand up for yourself and to convey the appropriate messages, leaving little chance for misunderstandings, while at the same time being sensitive and sympathetic to the needs, feelings and rights of other people.

Asserting yourself does not necessarily involve becoming aggressive, manipulative or heavy-handed or being offensive to friends and relatives. It should not make people dislike you or the boss fire you. What it does mean is learning to communicate effectively so that you are not intimidated by the salesman who is trying to sell you goods you don't want, or the total stranger who asks you for a date that you have no intention of agreeing to. It means you no longer give in to unreasonable demands and you are able to ask pertinent questions courteously and confidently. You do not have to suffer in silence because you feel unable to speak up, or

unwilling to stand up for your rights – by staying silent you are sowing the seeds for future headaches, high blood pressure and ulcers.

Self-assertion is the honest expression of your feelings and desires. It also entails taking responsibility for your own actions. It is the only way in which you can have your opinions heard, your claims met and your rights honoured.

How do you go about it?

The first step in learning to assert yourself is to identify those areas in which you have the most difficulty and least confidence. Situations in which you feel dependent, uncomfortable, awkward or frustrated might occur at home, where other members of your family make all the important decisions for you, or at work, where you find it impossible to ask for a rise or to refuse to do personal chores for your boss although they are not part of your job. Do you find it hard to start a conversation with a stranger at a party, or to complain to a shopkeeper for overcharging you or for selling you defective goods? It is a good idea to make a list of about ten situations in which you would like to be more assertive and self-confident.

Asserting yourself requires, above all, effective communication, and this starts with an effective dialogue with yourself. What do I want? What do I want to convey without sounding excessively demanding? How do I make it clear that this is very important to me? The next step is to realize that you are in control of yourself: you can decide what is important, what is acceptable and what is unsatisfactory. You are going to stop being dependent on others and worrying about how other people might judge, humiliate or criticize you.

What you say and how you say it are both part of a continuous process of communication, but even when you do not say anything your silence, gestures, movements and touch, all speak for you. Researchers estimate that more than half of the messages people send are conveyed non-verbally, by frowning, crossing your arms or legs, keeping a distance from others, looking at a clock, looking straight into someone's eyes (or not), blinking, staring, pointing a finger or banging a fist on the table.

Learning to assert yourself also involves raising your own self-esteem and feeling good about yourself. It sounds simple, but it can require a lot of time and persistent practice before you become really good at it. Even then, you may sometimes come up against some difficult situations when your courage may fail you.

ANGER MANAGEMENT

When Rip van Winkle got home after his 20-year sleep, he found that his ill-tempered wife had long since died of apoplexy (bursting of a blood vessel inside the brain, usually as the result of high blood pressure precipitating a stroke). It took a long time for science to realize the truth behind this folk wisdom – that the person who often explodes mentally is eventually at risk of exploding physically. More and more doctors now believe that anger, hostility and aggression are important factors in the development of high blood pressure and coronary heart disease.

Until recently, it was thought that it was only bottled-up anger which was harmful, and that anger that was outwardly expressed was all right. Anger can be expressed indirectly – by slamming doors or breaking a vase – or directly – by losing your temper, and making threats, hurling insults or striking out. However, many doctors now believe that rage, regardless of how effectively it is expressed, can boomerang and hit the victim you least of all intend – yourself.

ALTERING YOUR PERSPECTIVES

In Chapter 5, I discussed the coronary-prone Type A person, who is ambitious, impatient and competitive (see page 54). You may think that once a Type A, always a Type A, but it is in fact possible to change. A doctor who succeeded in changing his personality after having a heart attack made this comment: "After all, a sleeping tiger is just as gentle as a rabbit. Just don't challenge it by waking it up". Just as it can never be too late to stop smoking or drinking alcohol, so it is never too late to change a behaviour pattern that we know is a major factor in increasing the risk of heart attack.

The first step is to admit the existence of Type A behaviour. Unfortunately, four out of every five Type A subjects vehemently deny a Type A pattern of behaviour in themselves. Even if they might hesitantly admit it to their family doctors, they are most reluctant to do so to their spouses, their peers and, most of all, to their subordinates.

The second requirement is to believe that you can change this potentially destructive aspect of your personality. Most doctors have come across patients who, having survived a heart attack, have completely changed their lifestyle. They become calmer, delegate work and responsibility to others, and begin to enjoy some of life's simpler pleasures. Why not examine your behaviour patterns and attitudes right now? You do not have to wait for a crisis before you can change.

Puzzled by the fact that not everybody who is exposed to stress becomes ill, Suzanne Kobasa, a psychologist from Chicago, investigated groups of company executives, lawyers and army officers, and found that those who either resisted stress effectively or remained healthy in spite of stress resulting from life-events in the previous year, were disposed to commitment, control and challenge. Such a person is committed to his work, family and friends. He recognizes his goals and abilities, is realistic, resourceful, and knows where to go for help in times of need. He believes in his own ability to exert some control over his life and takes responsibility for what happens to him. He is prepared to accept challenges and to turn stressful life events into opportunities for personal growth rather than threats to his security. He responds to the unexpected with a sense of interest and exploration. He is naturally relaxed and more flexible in his attitudes.

ASSISTED RELAXATION

The impact of stress in our lives can be cushioned in two ways: by the strength and the number of supportive social relationships we have and by psychological assistance from breathing exercises, relaxation and meditation (see pages 158 to 165). The main sources of social support, in a decreasing order of importance, are: spouse or lover, other family members, friends, colleagues, health care personnel such as general practitioners, counsellors, health visitors or occupational nurses. Research studies have shown that death rates are lower in people with strong social relationships than in those who live lonely, isolated lives.

There are many examples showing the protective effect of social support. In a study of 10,000 Israeli civil servants, for instance, it was discovered that the incidence of angina among men who perceived their wives as loving and supportive was only half that of those who did not share this view. The health-sustaining role of a strong social support system also emerged from a study in California in which the lives of 4,700 men and women were followed for nine years. The death rate was highest in those men who were single, had few social contacts with friends or relatives, and were not church members. Marital status was not seen to make much difference to women, but, as with the men, close friendships, and membership of church and social clubs did mean a lower death rate.

There is even some evidence to show that pets provide some degree of protection against stress and illness. It has been reported, for example, that patients who own pets are more likely to recover from their heart attacks than those who do not. Physical contact is another symbol of caring and is considered to have healing powers. It is a pity that we do not touch and hug our friends and families more often. Why not decide to hug your partner and your children at least once a day?

THE IMPORTANCE OF RELAXATION

We all need to develop some sort of mechanism for relaxing and coping with stress. No one plan for coping will be satisfactory for everyone. Some people find that regular physical exercise has the desired effect (see Chapter 14), while others claim they need do nothing more than listen to music or allow themselves to become absorbed in a favourite hobby. But most of us are much more tense than we realize and real relaxation, both mental and physical, means much more than simply sitting down and "taking it easy" for a moment.

Relaxation is a skill, like driving a car, and it has to be learned until, again like driving a car, it becomes second nature. There are several forms of auto, of self-induced, relaxation, which anyone can learn and practise. They require only a few minutes of daily practice, and many people find them of tremendous benefit. Popular methods include deep breathing exercises (see page 158), deep muscle relaxation (see page 159), meditation (see page 163) and autogenic training (see page 166).

The stress response includes irregular breathing, the tensing of muscles in readiness for "fight or flight" and inner feelings of turmoil and panic. It makes sense, then, that regular breathing, for example, makes you feel calm and composed; physical relaxation will not only reduce physical tension but also calm the mind; and a totally relaxed mind, which may be aided by meditation, is incompatible with the stress response.

THE BENEFITS OF RELAXATION

When you are deeply relaxed, through meditation for example, your oxygen consumption – or the rate at which the body burns up energy – will decrease dramatically. It takes about five or six hours' sleep to achieve this low level of oxygen consumption and, since sleep is very recuperative, you can appreciate the benefits of deep rest which can be achieved by only a few minutes practising a relaxation technique.

Cardiac output – or the amount of blood passing through the heart every minute – also falls markedly if you are relaxed, which indicates a reduction in the heart's workload. The heart can never rest completely, but working in continuous overdrive, for whatever

reason – prolonged exercise or emotion, for example – can be harmful. The heart needs time to recuperate every now and again and it seems that short periods of deep relaxation are the perfect way of achieving this.

It helps the body use oxygen

Your body needs a continuous supply of energy to keep it working. This energy is obtained from the food you eat, but in order to burn up the food and produce energy, you need oxygen. When they are both adequate, the body machine runs smoothly; the fuel is completely used up and waste products, such as carbon dioxide and water, are eliminated.

If, however, you need to use energy faster than you can supply oxygen to burn the food, or fuel, it will break down only partially and intermediate products, like lactate, or lactic acid, accumulate in the body. For example, if you climb stairs too rapidly, you may start to feel breathless and you may also develop a pain in your calves. As soon as you take in enough oxygen, your breathing returns to normal and the ache in your calf muscles disappears; the lactate breaks down into water and carbon dioxide, both of which can now be eliminated.

There is evidence to suggest that deep relaxation reduces the concentration of lactate in the blood. This is particularly important because lactate levels are at their highest when a person is in a state of anxiety. In fact, researchers have now shown that an anxiety state can actually be induced by infusing lactate into the bloodstream using an intravenous drip. Lactate levels are high in about a third of people with high blood pressure.

It retunes the vital functions

Stress causes us to break out in a sweat, the presence of which prepares the skin for the passage of an electrical current, which can be measured on a meter – this is the principle on which lie detectors are based. When you relax, on the other hand, the skin's resistance to a current increases and the deeper the relaxation, the greater the skin's resistance to an electrical current.

Relaxation also makes breathing become slower and abdominal, or dia-phragmatic, which is the most efficient way of breathing (see page 158). And the brainwave pattern becomes more harmoniously synchronized suggesting that the left side of the brain works in tune with the right and the front works in tune with the back.

RELAXATION TRAINING

Over the last 15 years, I have developed a programme of training which includes stress management techniques, breath-ing exercises, deep muscle relaxation, biofeedback (see page 165), and a form of yogic meditation for people who have high blood pressure or who are at risk of developing heart disease because of other risk factors. Learning and regu-larly practising these skills has proved successful in reducing blood pressure in several controlled experiments.

In one such experiment, nearly 200 "high risk" patients were randomly allo-cated to treatment and control groups. Patients in both groups were given the usual advice to stop smoking, to reduce fat in their diet, and to make sure that their blood pressure did not get out of control by having it checked regularly and by following their doctor's advice. In addition, the treatment group was trained in breathing exercises, deep muscle relaxation and meditation aided by biofeedback. Four years later, blood pressure was significantly lower in the treatment group than in the control group. There were also more people in

the control group who reported angina and other complications of high blood pressure. When their ECG's had been analysed by someone who did not know how the groups were divided, it was found that there were five new cases of coronary heart disease in the control group, compared with only one in the treatment group. And there was one fatal heart attack in the control group.

People who relax regularly, both mentally and physically, also adjust more quickly to a stressful environment and are less likely to react adversely to it. This does not, however, mean that they are any less vigilant or that their senses are in any way dulled. In fact, it has been shown that those who practise regular relaxation have an improved memory, heightened sensory aware-ness, and faster reactions to potentially dangerous situations. In one experi-ment, for example, it was shown that clarity and acuity of hearing were greatly improved after deep physio-logical rest.

One of my patients, a 78-year-old woman with high blood pressure, followed my relaxation course, and was asked by a television interviewer how she had benefited. Among various things, she mentioned that her vision had improved considerably and that she was now wearing her older, weaker glasses. This was the first time that I had heard this sort of response and no one was more surprised than me. I was also sceptical until I heard similar reports from other therapists.

Another of my patients said, after a 20-minute relaxation session, "Every-thing is so clear. It is as if someone had taken my brain out, scrubbed it and put it back again!" Indeed, people's learn-ing ability seems to improve and better academic performances after relaxation training have been reported.

Relaxation programmes at work

When companies have introduced relaxation or meditation breaks for their workforce, they have reported both improved performance and high job satisfaction. My own team carried out a relaxation training programme in an electronics company, for people we identified as being at risk from future heart disease. We were able to report a significantly greater reduction in both blood pressure and coronary heart disease in the group that was trained in relaxation than in the people who were merely advised to change their diet and stop smoking. In addition to this, more people in the relaxation group reported better powers of concentration, better relationships with their families and colleagues, better mental and physical health, more energy, a better social life and even a better sex life.

Other benefits

Occasionally, patients have claimed to feel less depressed, more tolerant, more trusting and more loving following a course in relaxation or meditation. Some people have been able to give up tranquillizers, sleeping pills, alcohol, cigarettes, marijuana, cannabis, and even hard drugs such as heroin.

Relaxation is certainly a wonderful way of putting yourself to bed. Several of my patients tell me something like this: "Last night I couldn't sleep so I started doing the deep muscle relaxation you taught me. I can't remember anything after the left knee!"

RELAXATION PROGAMME

Over the next few pages I describe the various techniques that I make use of in my relaxation programme – breathing exercises, deep muscle relaxation, meditation and biofeedback – as well as a few other techniques such as autogenic training and massage. If you want to build up your own relaxation programme I suggest that in the first week you practise the breathing exercises (see page 159), in the second week do the breathing and deep muscle relaxation (see page 159). By the third week you should add the visualization at the end of deep muscle relaxation (see page 162). By the fourth week you should begin to include meditation into your relaxation routine.

Everyday relaxation

In order to mitigate the effect of every-day stress, you also need to relax generally and not just look upon relaxation as a ritual performed once or twice a day. Relaxation practised briefly and often, ensures that tension never builds up to the degree that you feel really upset, angry or frustrated.

Try the following for a start. If you drive, every time you stop at a red traffic light, release your grip on the steering wheel, take a deep breath and relax. It doesn't matter whether this is for three seconds or 30. Another thing you can do is to take a deep breath and compose yourself before you pick up the telephone. You will notice the difference in your interaction with the person at the other end of the line; you will be less impulsive, calmer and more thoughtful. If you are one of those people who live by their watch, stick a little red dot on the face of your wrist watch, so that every time you are under pressure and you look at your watch, you will be reminded to calm down. You can work out a variety of different ways in which you can remind yourself to build these mini relaxation techniques into your daily life – all of which are tailor-made for you. Notice which situations make you tense, then work out some signs to remind yourself to relax.

BREATHING EXERCISES

Breathing is essential to life. Life begins with a breath and stops when a person has taken his last breath. Breathing is involuntary, by which I mean that you do not have to make a conscious effort to breathe. It is automatic because it is controlled, like all our other internal functions, by the autonomic, or involuntary, nervous system.

However, breathing is also unique in that it can be consciously controlled through special breathing exercises, which override the autonomic nervous system. Since we breathe between 16,000 and 20,000 times a day, breathing exercises are a very powerful tool.

Although breathing is one of man's vital functions, it is little understood. Since it is automatic, it is a reliable reflection of our state of mind. For example, people tend to breathe rapidly and often, using only the upper part of the chest, when they are in a state of high anxiety. Depressed people sigh frequently. Anxious people talk at the peak of inhalation, while depressed people talk at the end of exhalation.

HOW YOU SHOULD BREATHE

There are two distinct ways of breathing: costal (meaning "of the ribs") and abdominal breathing.

Costal breathing

This type of breathing is characterized by an outward, upward movement of the chest. It is useful during vigorous exercise but it is quite inappropriate for ordinary, everyday activity.

Abdominal breathing

The principal muscle involved in abdominal breathing is the diaphragm, a strong dome-shaped sheet of muscle, that separates the chest cavity from the abdomen. When you breathe in, the diaphragm contracts and pushes downwards, causing the abdomen to relax. In this position, the lungs expand, creating a partial vacuum which draws air in. When you breathe out, the diaphragm

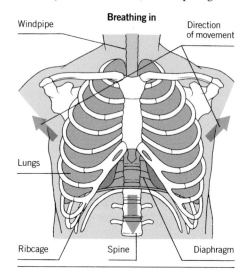

Breathing in

Windpipe

Direction of movement

Lungs

Ribcage   Spine   Diaphragm

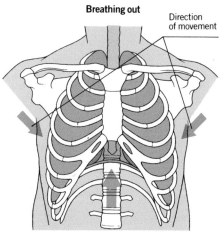

Breathing out

Direction of movement

How we breathe
Air flows into the lungs when the diaphragm decends and the rib cage expands to increase the capacity of the lungs. When the diaphragm relaxes and the ribs fall, air is pushed out of the lungs.

BREATHING CORRECTLY

1 Lie on your back with your feet a comfortable distance apart and gently close your eyes. Place one hand on your abdomen to feel the movement of the abdominal muscles, and place the other hand on your chest to check that there is little or no movement here.

2 Inhale and exhale slowly, smoothly, and deeply through the nostrils. There should be no noise, no jerks and no pauses in the breath. To exaggerate the normal breathing process you can consciously pull in the abdominal muscles when you exhale. If you find this movement difficult, push your abdominal muscles in gently with your hands as you exhale. When you inhale, be aware of the abdominal wall pushing out.

3 Practise this method of deep breathing for between three and five minutes a day until you clearly understand the movement of the diaphragm and the abdominal muscles. The body is designed to breathe diaphragmatically and it should gradually become a natural function, whether you are standing, sitting or lying down.

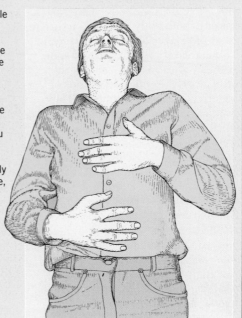

relaxes, the abdomen contracts and expels air containing carbon dioxide.

Diaphragmatic breathing is the most important tool available for stress management. It promotes a natural, even movement of breath which both strengthens the nervous system and relaxes the body. It is the most efficient method of breathing, using the minimum effort in return for the maximum oxygen. It has three important beneficial effects on the body:

● It fills the lungs completely, providing the body with sufficient oxygen.
● It forces carbon dioxide, the waste product of respiration, out of the lungs. When you breathe shallowly, some carbon dioxide may remain in the lungs, and can cause fatigue and nervousness.
● The up-and-down motion of the diaphragm gently massages the abdominal organs. This increases the circulation to these organs, which makes them function more efficiently.

DEEP MUSCLE RELAXATION

Each time one of your muscles contracts, thousands of impulses travel along the nerves to the brain. There is also some evidence to suggest that the part of the brain which controls blood pressure and emotions, the hypothalamus, becomes highly charged when it is bombarded with all the sensory stimulations to which it is constantly exposed.

It is possible to cut down drastically on the sensory impulses travelling to the brain simply by lying down, closing your eyes, learning not to be distracted by external noises, and then deeply relaxing your entire body. The result is amazing: both body and mind return to a state of balance or recuperative rest.

Such relaxation should occur spontaneously after any activity but, unfortunately, the endless demands of modern life often prevent this. The result is a continuous state of stress, which can eventually culminate in a stress disorder. You need to learn the art of letting go and allowing your body's restorative ability to take over.

The aim of deep muscle relaxation

The relaxation technique described left and opposite will help you to release habitual, often unconscious, tension and replace it with a beneficial state of relaxation. It starts with simple deep breathing, followed by relaxation of all the muscles in the body and then by relaxation of the mind by detachment and visualization. The whole process lasts 15 to 20 minutes. If you practise twice a day for a week or two, you will find that your level of relaxation deepens considerably and you may even find that you fall asleep. Your mind may still be restless, however, in which case you will benefit from progressing to the next stage which is meditation (see page 163). Meditation calms the restless mind and also helps you to remain awake, yet profoundly relaxed. This is

important since the aim of becoming relaxed is to control blood pressure while still allowing you to carry on with your normal daily activities. If you still find it difficult to stay awake, practise relaxation sitting up.

HOW TO PRACTICE DEEP MUSCLE RELAXATION

Read the following instructions several times or better still, ask a friend to read them to you slowly in a low monotonous voice while you follow them. Alternatively, record the instructions on a tape recorder and then practise while you listen to it.

Start with stage one and add further stages as you become more proficient. However many stages you complete, always prepare yourself as described below and come out of relaxation following the instructions.

Preparation

Lie flat on your back on a firm bed or folded blanket on the floor; make sure your head, trunk and legs are in a straight line. Keep your knees together and relax your legs. Allow your feet to flop loosely, with your toes pointing outwards. If you are not used to lying flat on the floor, you may find this uncomfortable to start with; if so, use a small pillow under your head and a folded towel or cushion behind your knees or under your lower back. Alternatively, lie back in a reclining chair.

Relax your jaw, your teeth must not be clenched, and relax your shoulders. If you are lying on the floor, let your shoulders drop down to the floor. Your arms should fall away from your body with the palms facing the ceiling and the fingers curling naturally. Close your eyes and, as you breathe out, let your body sink into the floor or chair. Now you are ready to relax deeply.

TIPS FOR DEEP MUSCLE RELAXATION

■ Do not practise on a full stomach; allow at least one and a half hours after you have eaten a light meal.
■ Make sure that you are comfortable, warm and have no constricting clothes, ties or belts.
■ Remove your shoes, and, if you wear them spectacles or contact lenses.

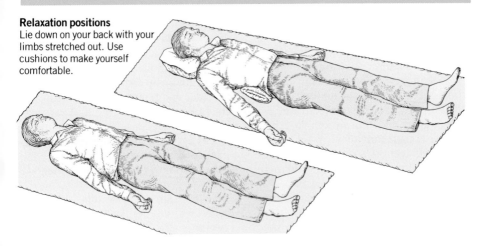

Relaxation positions
Lie down on your back with your limbs stretched out. Use cushions to make yourself comfortable.

Stage one: breathing

Very slowly fill your lungs, starting at the diaphragm and working right up to the top of the chest, then very slowly breathe out. After a few breaths, your breathing will be normal and regular. Breathe in and out gently and rhythmically. Don't force your breath. Don't try to make it slow. Just keep to your own rhythm. Concentrate your mind on the difference in temperature between the air you inhale and the air you exhale.

Stage two: relaxation

The next stage involves consciously relaxing each part of the body in turn. Relaxation means the complete absence of movement, since even the slightest movement would mean that some of your muscles are contracting. It is also the opposite of holding any part rigid Concentrate on the part of the body you are relaxing. In this way you will discover the interlinking of mind and body and how one can affect the other.

● First take your mind to your right foot and relax your toes, instep, heel and ankle; now move your attention slowly up your leg and relax your calf, knee, thigh and hip. Feel all your muscles becoming relaxed and limp. Become aware of every part of your right leg and relax them as deeply as you can.

● Take your mind to your left foot and repeat the process, working up the leg. Let all the tension ease away and enjoy the sensation of relaxation throughout.

● Next concentrate on your right hand and relax the fingers, thumb, palm and wrist. Move your attention up to your forearm, then on to your elbow, upper arm and shoulder and feel every muscle becoming limp. Relax as deeply as you can. Fix your attention on the sensation of total relaxation in your right arm.

● Now become aware of your left hand. Relax your fingers, thumb, palm and wrist. Slowly move your attention up to your forearm, elbow, upper arm and shoulder. Let all the tension drain away from the muscles. Feel the relaxation and limpness throughout your left arm.

● Now concentrate on the base of your spine. Work your way up the spine, vertebra by vertebra, and relax each vertebra and the muscles on either side of the spine into the floor. Feel your back merging with the floor. Now relax the muscles of your upper back. Release all the tension from them. Relax your neck. Let all the muscles in your neck relax completely, first at the front of the neck then at the back. Let your head rest gently and feel all the muscles in the back of your neck relaxing. Just let them go and carry on letting them go.

• Now concentrate on your chin and relax it. Relax your jaw and let it drop down slightly so that your teeth are slightly apart and your lips just touching. Relax your tongue. Now relax your cheeks and feel them relaxing. Relax the muscles around your eyes and feel them becoming heavy and very relaxed. There is no tension in your eyes, nor in the muscles around your eyes. They are in a state of complete relaxation. Now relax your forehead. Just let all the tension release from the muscles of your forehead. Feel all the muscles in your face relaxing. There is no tension in your facial muscles at all. Now relax your scalp. Feel the relaxation in the muscles around your head.

• Now relax your chest. Every time you breathe out, relax a little more. Let your body sink into the floor, a little more each time. Let all the muscles, nerves and organs in your chest relax completely. Now, relax your stomach muscles. Let all the muscles, nerves and organs in your stomach relax totally.

• Your body is completely and totally relaxed. Keep it relaxed and concentrate on your breathing. Feel the cool air going in and the warm air coming out of your nostrils. Stay in the relaxed position for a few minutes.

Coming out of relaxation

Take a deep breath and feel the energy coming back into your arms; move your fingers slightly. Take another deep breath and feel the energy returning to your legs; move your toes slightly. Gradually stretch your arms and legs. Next open your eyes slowly without reacting to the light. Slowly sit up, and continue the feeling of peace within you.

DETACHMENT WITH CREATIVE VISUALIZATION

When you feel comfortable with deep muscle relaxation, probably after a week or two, you can progress to the next stage and relax your mind with detachment and visualization. Learning to become detached will allow you to be objective when you are confronted with a particular problem. Visualization teaches you how to conjure up a mental picture of your goal and to retain this image long enough to be able to furnish it with creative energy so that eventually it becomes a reality.

The technique outlined below is not a mere ritual, it has a very real application in everyday life. You will retain a positive outlook on life even after you come out of this utterly relaxed state. This attitude helps you to visualize and achieve your goals.

Visualization can help you to achieve anything you want in life on a mental, spiritual or physical level. Most people have an idea of something they want, for example, to get a new job, or to develop a relationship with someone. You must bear in mind that you cannot control other people's behaviour through this process. However relaxation opens your mind and helps you to become more receptive to others, by doing this you at least dissolve barriers and allow them to be more natural. At first you should set yourself simple tasks. If you can achieve these simple goals, you will find that your confidence gradually increases until you feel that nothing is impossible. Our present goal is to create a peaceful atmosphere (see below).

Becoming detached

Practise the breathing exercises and deep muscle relaxation described earlier. When you are totally relaxed, continue as follows:

• Let your mind become very, very still. Untie the knots of tension. Try not to concentrate on any particular thought. Let your thoughts just float by. Take a step back from them so you are only observing them. Let the thoughts come and go without lingering on any particular one. Let yourself become detached from your mind, so that you are still in the state of total relaxation.

• Now picture a calm and beautiful lake in your mind. The sun is shining down on the lake. Your mind is like that lake. It must be very, very still. Experience a feeling of spaciousness. The lake is so still that you can see right through it – through the lake into a large open space, with the sun still beating down into that space. So there is warmth, and there is peace, there is calm and there is joy. These are the only feelings that you can experience: feelings of peace, of calm, of joy, of warmth and of energy.

• A thought would disturb this state of peace. You can control your thoughts at will. You are master. You want to keep the feeling of openness, of spaciousness, of light, warmth and energy. Concentrate on these feelings; experience them; go into them; surrender yourself totally to these experiences and feelings. Feel wave after wave of relaxation pouring over your whole being.

• Stay with the image for five minutes and then come out of the relaxed state as described for deep muscle relaxation.

MEDITATION

The word meditation in its common, colloquial sense implies thinking about a problem, whereas used with reference to therapy, it means bringing the mind under control in order to liberate it from all intrusive thoughts. In this context it is considered to be the fourth stage in the building up of your programme of complete relaxation.

Meditation has been practised in India and Asia for centuries, it is, for example, central to the yogi's way of life. Various forms of meditation have been incorporated into many religions and cultures for example, Christian prayer, Jewish meditation, Islamic sufi, Chinese tao, Japanese zen and so on.

Recently, however, many people in the medical profession, have recognized that meditation can be used, without any religious connotation, as a form of therapy to relieve stress and promote health. There is now ample evidence to suggest that meditation does have significant psychological and physiological benefits, including a positive reduction in heart rate, respiration, skin conductivity and blood pressure.

What meditation involves

Meditation entails adopting a comfortable position – which is usually sitting, although it can also be lying or standing – in a quiet room, taking a physically relaxed and mentally passive attitude, and dwelling single-mindedly on just one thing. This can be an object, such as fruit or a flower; an idea, a mental picture or a phrase or word called a "mantra"; it can mean turning inwards on your own thought processes; or it can be some bodily generated rhythm such as breathing. This leaves you free to choose whatever method best suits your particular intellectual and emotional make-up.

The aim of meditation

Ultimately, the aim is to discipline your mind to concentrate on a single thing.

Voluntary concentration on one subject can not only help you to see and think about that subject with great clarity, but it also brings all the different ideas and memories associated with that subject into your mind. As deeper levels of concentration are achieved, the whole process of meditation becomes more intimate and compelling.

Like deep muscle relaxation and visualization, meditation is more than just a ritual, it has many practical applications. It is well known that the mind that can hold an idea, can become held by it. For example, if you constantly tell yourself that you are a failure and that you are inferior, you will eventually come to believe it. Meditation can focus the mind and turn this power of the subconscious into something more positive which can then be used to build up your character rather than destroy it. It can help you feel more complete and closer to yourself and therefore help you to relate to others more easily.

Just as there are different objects upon which we can meditate, there are many different ways in which the goal of

HOW TO MEDITATE

■ Practise regularly. Meditation is most beneficial if you practise it for about ten to 20 minutes twice a day.

■ Avoid distractions. Meditate in a quiet room where there is a minimal level of noise, light and activity.

■ Be comfortable. Make sure the room is warm, wear loose clothes and empty your bladder and bowel beforehand. Do not meditate for at least two hours after a meal.

■ Meditate sitting down. The classic Eastern posture is the yogic lotus, half lotus or cross-legged position but these are by no means essential. Another method is to sit on a comfortable upright chair, with your back straight but not rigid, your body comfortable and still. The tip of your nose should be in line with your navel, and your eyes closed.

■ Breathe gently. Take quiet, smooth gentle breaths through the nostrils and take the air right down to the abdomen (see page 159).

■ Relax completely from your feet upwards as described on pages 160-162.

■ Concentrate your mind on one thing. The easiest, most available thing is the rhythm of your own breath, which you can follow by counting your exhalations. Count from one to ten, then start at one again. Alternatively, you can choose a physical object, such as a fruit, flower or candle which you gaze at, your eyes only just open, for a few minutes, then close your eyes and view the "after image" in your mind. When the image disappears open your eyes again, gaze at the object, close them again, and so on. After a while you won't need to look at a real object at all but will be able to meditate entirely by visualizing your chosen object in your mind.

You can also choose a "mantra" – a word or phrase which you repeat mentally. You can either select a neutral word like "om" or "one", or a word like "love" or "peace" which has pleasant contemplative associations. Alternatively, listen to a piece of music or to the sound of the sea lapping against the shore; or concentrate on the smell of freshly cut grass after you have mown the lawn. Try several methods until you find the one that suits you best.

■ Remain passive. Observe a passive and relaxed attitude towards any distractions. Thoughts are bound to flit in and out of your mind – what you're having for supper, what's on the television, something you forgot to do earlier. Every time that your mind wanders, bring it back easily and effortlessly to the object of your meditation, always remaining relaxed and passive. Accept that it is inevitable that your mind will wander, don't be discouraged and don't keep thinking about how you're doing. As you get more practised, so your mind will wander less frequently.

■ Come out of meditation very slowly and gently as described for deep muscle relaxation (see page 162).

meditation can be approached. For some people it is approached through the intellect – the belief that wisdom can be developed to the point of transcendence; for some, it is through the emotions – as in the Christian surrender to God; for others it is through the body – as in the physical postures of Hatha yoga, the Chinese movement therapy, t'ai chi or the Western Alexander technique; and for yet others it is attained through action. The latter can mean concentrating on jogging or even washing up to the exclusion of everything else in the external world, or perhaps the Oriental martial arts of aikido and karate, or rug weaving as practised in the Moslem sufi tradition.

Whichever way you choose to meditate, you may well find that it is more difficult than you imagined. You may be surprised at how unruly and undisciplined your mind proves to be, but this is not at all unusual and you should not be put off by it. Accept it positively and objectively and, with practice, patience, and perseverance, you will acquire the technique.

BIOFEEDBACK

The concept of biofeedback is a major scientific breakthrough which enables us to monitor the body's inner, and thus hidden, responses to relaxation therapy. Those bodily functions over which we have direct control, such as walking and talking, are supplied by a voluntary nervous system; while those over which we do not have direct control, such as the heartbeat and blood pressure, are supplied by the autonomic, or involuntary, nervous system.

The idea of the group of scientists who pioneered biofeedback was that it might be possible to learn to control the involuntary functions if only we could actually see or hear them. Accordingly, they developed electronic instruments to which a person can be connected painlessly by electrodes and which literally "feed back" information about various internal biological functions. The functions which can be monitored in this way include heart rate, blood pressure, electrical resistance of the skin and thus sweat gland activity, muscle tension, skin temperature and brainwave pattern, which is shown on a special electroencephalograph (EEG).

How does it work?

Biofeedback encourages you to exert a certain control over your body's internal functions by making you conscious of what is happening inside your body as it responds to various subjective or behavioural stages. If you succeed in

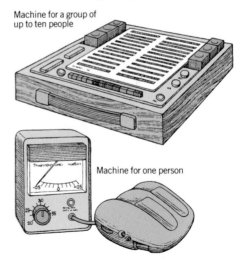

Machine for a group of up to ten people

Machine for one person

Biofeedback machines
There are several different types of machine and they supply the feedback in several different ways: by sounds, such as clicks and tones, by lights, and by the rise and fall of a needle on a chart.

bringing about any inner change, bio-feedback informs you of it. By trial and error and with the help of a therapist, you can learn to control a particular function. Knowledge of your success will reinforce your ability to learn.

Where do you find this therapy?
Biofeedback machines are easily available but can be very expensive and are not generally recommended for home

use. Under the guidance of a therapist qualified in the use of the biofeedback machines, however, this therapy can be of tremendous use as an aid to learning how to relax. The most usual way to use it therefore, is in conjunction with other therapies, such as yoga or relaxation. I usually use it to measure sweat gland activity, in conjunction with breathing exercises, relaxation and meditation, for patients with high blood pressure.

OTHER RELAXATION THERAPIES

There are many different types of relaxation training. So far, I have discussed the methods which I myself favour and which I use for my own patients, but there are several others.

PROGRESSIVE MUSCLE RELAXATION
Progressive muscle relaxation, or PMR, is similar in many ways to deep muscle relaxation (see page 159) except that instead of simply relaxing each group of muscles in turn, you first tense each group of mu˜les before relaxing it. This has been found to reduce both the pulse rate and blood pressure. Tensing muscles can, however, first increase blood pressure quite dramatically, albeit only temporarily, so I generally recommend deep muscle relaxation. It is, though, perfectly safe for people who do not have high blood pressure and some people, particularly those of an anxious disposition, actually prefer it.

What you do
● First, loosen any constricting items of clothing and take off your shoes.
● Lie down or sit in a comfortable upright chair and distribute your weight evenly; do not cross your arms or legs.
● Close your eyes.

● Take a deep breath and let it out again slowly. Breathe regularly and naturally, in as passive a way as you can.
● Make a fist with your right hand and tighten the upper arm as if you were going to lift a heavy weight. Do not move your arm but hold it tight for about five to seven seconds. Focus on the feeling of tension.
● Release the tension and breathe out, letting go of more and more tension as you exhale. Let your arm relax for 20-30 seconds. Pause for a minute and focus on the new feeling of relaxation. Repeat with the opposite arm.

When you start PMR, practise on only one or two groups of muscles in the first few sessions until you have mastered the technique of tensing and relaxing. Then you can progress to tightening and relaxing all ten groups of muscles in the following order: right arm; left arm; forehead; eyes, cheeks, nose and jaw; lips and tongue; neck; chest, back and shoulders; abdomen and buttocks; right leg; left leg.

AUTOGENICS
Autogenic training is a series of mental exercises which switch off the body's "fight or flight" mechanism and switch on its system of rest and relaxation. It is

called autogenic because it is based on self, or auto, suggestion. The result is similar to that of meditation.

What does it comprise?

Autogenic training consists of six basic exercises, including imagining that your arms and legs are heavy; your arms and legs are warm; your breathing is calm and regular; your forehead is cool; your heartbeat is slow and regular; and your solar plexus is warm.

Autogenics can be self-taught though it is better to learn them under the supervision of a qualified teacher as they can sometimes cause adverse reactions, such as palpitations or a rise in blood pressure. You will normally have an eight-week course consisting of one hour's instruction per week and you will be asked to perform the exercises twice or three times a day. You can practise anywhere, for between 20 and 30 minutes twice a day, or for between three and five minutes several times a day.

What you will do

Sit, either on an easy or upright chair, or lie down on your back. Do not cross your arms or legs. You will then be taught the first exercise. For example, you will be asked to think about your right arm and say to yourself "My right arm is heavy". Repeat this several times, after a few seconds' pause each time. You will then proceed to your left arm, both arms, right leg, left leg, both legs, neck, shoulders.

At the end of each session you make fists, tense your arms, bend them and take a deep breath, then stretch your arms. Pause for a few minutes before you stand up and resume your normal, everyday activities.

MASSAGE

Being massaged is enjoyable and relaxing. The human touch brings feelings of warmth and being cared for which greatly increase our sense of well-being. Massage also stimulates the circulation, which both brings a fresh supply of fuel to all parts of the body and removes accumulated toxic wastes. It is therefore also therapeutic.

The art of giving a massage lies in knowing which part of the hand to use and how much pressure to apply for each movement and this can only be learned by practising. It is important that your hands are kept in constant contact with your partner's body and that you maintain a regular rhythm. Stopping and starting, or lifting your hands in the middle, interrupts the rhythm and destroys the effect. Overleaf are step-by-step instructions for giving someone a massage using some of the best-known massage techniques: stroking, pummeling, kneading, circular pressure and percussion movements. It is hoped that it will inspire you to look deeper into the subject, either by reading a more detailed book on massage or, better still, by attending a short course. For details of organizations, see Useful Addresses, page 187.

Self-massage

It is very difficult to relax while massaging yourself as some of your muscles will be working and therefore inevitably tense. You can, however, massage any specific areas that feel tense, such as your scalp, the back of your neck, your temples, shoulders, hands, lower back, calves and feet. You can adapt any of the movements given overleaf.

GIVING A MASSAGE

Ask your partner to lie face down, naked or wearing only underwear, on a blanket or towel, either on a large table or on the floor. Do not use a bed, it would be too soft and most of the pressure would be absorbed by the mattress. Make sure that the room is warm and only softly lit.

Although not essential, it is helpful to use some sort of lubricant, such as a body cream or baby oil. The deep, long stroking movements used at the start of the massage will help to spread this lubricant all over the body, and will relax and soothe your partner before you start the firmer strokes.

1 Start off by placing your thumbs on either side of your partner's spine and moving the palms of your hands upwards and outwards using large circular stroking movements. These movements should be smooth and rhythmical; apply firm pressure as you work towards your partner's heart and more gentle pressure as you work away from the heart.

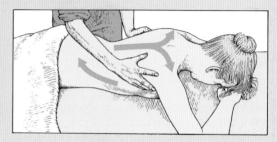

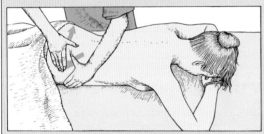

2 Knead the buttocks and sides using rolling, pressing and squeezing movements as if you are working bread dough; this stimulates the circulation and encourages relaxation. Then, place one hand on top of the other and use the heel of the lower hand to apply pressure to the buttocks.

3 Place your thumbs on either side of the spine at the base of the neck, make deep strokes up to the top and, moving your hands to her side, glide back down to the base again. Follow this with friction at the base of the skull and then make tapping movements on the shoulders with your fingers as if playing the piano.

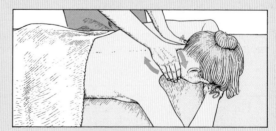

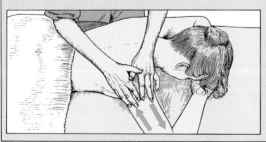

4 Apply pressure and kneading movements around the shoulder-blades, and continue stroking along the shoulders to the upper arms. Stroke and knead all areas including the hands and fingers; using only your thumbs and fingers when working on small areas. Finish with progressively lighter stroking movements over the whole arm.

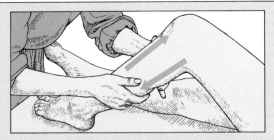

5 Ask your partner to turn over onto her back. Stroke the whole leg or specific areas, such as the calves, knees, ankles with deep or light movements according to the fleshiness of the area you are working on.

6 Use both hands to stroke each foot in turn, working on the instep, arch and then toes. Then, using your thumbs, apply small circular pressure movements to each toe and the soles of the feet.

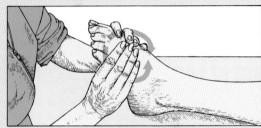

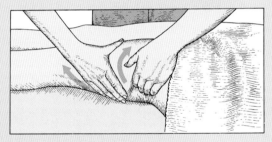

7 Then work on the calves and thighs. Knead them as above and pummel them with the fleshy side of loosely clenched fists applying first one fist and then the other. If applied gently, this is useful for releasing tension in the thighs. Stroke the calves and thighs then the whole leg. Finish with progressively lighter strokes.

8 Stroke up the abdomen and glide your hands down the sides. Knead the hips, sides and — lightly — the stomach. Cup your hands and place them on the stomach for a minute.

9 Work on the face and the neck. Start with deep strokes on the forehead, working from the centre to the temples. Repeat below the eyebrows.

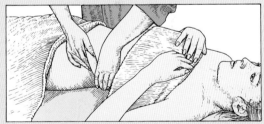

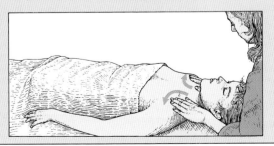

10 Cup your hands under the chin, stroke up to the ears. Move onto the hinge of the jaw, supporting the head with one hand while applying pressure strokes with the other. Then give deep strokes from the jaw to the collarbone, working the thumbs on the fleshy part of the neck. Finish by stroking the forehead with your thumbs.

14
Keeping fit

Physical exercise is as necessary to life as water, food and sunlight – it is indispensable if we wish to stay healthy, strong and agile.

The human body was designed for the active life our ancestors led, running to catch food and fighting off predators. Modern city life makes none of these demands on the body and it is not surprising that many people become stiff, flabby and fat.

You may be tempted to think that as long as you can drive a car or take the bus or train, why walk? If you can take an elevator, why climb stairs? But if you do not exercise, your muscles will atrophy, joints will stiffen, your circulation will become sluggish, you will get depressed, and you will be short of breath on the slightest exertion. Premature heart disease is the biggest price to be paid for our sedentary life.

There are innumerable reasons for taking regular exercise. On the following pages I describe some of the most important, and suggest some exercises.

A FITTER HEART

The role of exercise in the prevention of coronary heart disease has been established by a number of long-term observations. Research has demonstrated, for example, that those who take regular, vigorous exercise have a much lower chance of having a heart attack; and that if they do have one, they are more likely to survive it. Exercise strengthens the heart, and the fitter heart is more stable, with less likelihood of developing heart irregularities (rhythm disturbance) or sudden failure.

Exactly how exercise protects against heart disease is less clear. Heart disease is attributable to many risk factors (see Chapters 4 and 5) and exercise is believed to protect the heart indirectly by reducing many of them. It certainly helps reduce obesity, for example, and there is much circumstantial evidence to suggest that it also reduces high blood pressure, perhaps by making the blood vessels more supple and elastic, though its role here has not as yet been substantiated. And it also seems to make the arteries more resistant to atheromatous plaque.

Another risk factor which is thought to be influenced by exercise is the level of fats, or lipids, in the blood. The latest investigations suggest that exercise may actually help to reduce the level of harmful triglycerides and low density lipoproteins (LDL), while at the same time it seems to raise the level of beneficial high density lipoproteins (HDL), (see page 63).

Exercise is also believed to improve the coronary circulation. As the heart, like any other muscle which receives regular exercise, grows stronger, so the capacity of the lungs increases and the heart pumps more blood with each beat. As the amount of blood that the body needs remains static, so the heart beats more slowly, but more efficiently, both when exercising and at rest. More work can therefore be done at the expense of less effort, and with a lower pulse rate. A low resting pulse (below 72 beats per minute) is indicative of heart/lung, or cardiovascular, efficiency.

Exercise balances body and mind

Modern living is very competitive at all levels; anger, frustration and hostility have become part of our daily life. This causes the release of stress hormones adrenaline, noradrenaline, cortisol and serotonin, and the mobilization of fats and sugars in the blood. This leads to a spiral whereby, as you become more depressed, you seek out more stress and excitement or artificial stimulants. This causes yet more stress hormones to be released and more fats and sugars are mobilized. Exercise uses up these substances, thereby balancing the mind and body. In addition, gentle rhythmic exercise such as swimming, jogging, cycling and walking, is a very good way to release tension because mind and body both relax into the soothing rhythm of the exercise.

BENEFITS OF EXERCISE

There are many advantages of taking regular exercise. Some of the most important are as follows:

- It prevents coronary artery disease
- It increases cardiovascular efficiency
- It reduces the risk of a heart attack
- It tones up the muscles and improves your figure
- It helps you relax
- It helps you sleep better
- It makes you more alert
- It regulates your appetite
- It generates vitality and confidence
- It improves the digestion
- It increases physical strength
- It keeps the joints supple
- It maintains a good, erect posture
- It improves mental concentration
- It promotes your mental and spiritual development
- It may improve your intellectual capacity
- It makes child bearing less painful
- It lessens the likelihood of sedentary diseases such as rheumatism, arthritis, diabetes, backache and depression; it is also known to help asthmatics

Exercise lessens the chances of your developing sedentary disease and can improve intellectual capacity. In a research project carried out in a French school to study the effects of regular exercise, the time given to physical education was increased by a third. The results showed that the academic performance of the students increased and the amount of illness decreased.

THE "S" FACTORS

Before you embark on any exercise programme, or sporting activity, it is very important to consider the five so-called "S" factors – safety, suppleness, stamina, strength and satisfaction – as described on the following pages. This is even more important if you are suffering from coronary artery disease.

SAFETY

First of all, make sure that you choose a suitable activity for your age and ability.

171

Join classes where you can get expert advice or read books that will give you the relevant background information. You must also have the correct equipment, if it is required.

People often have sudden bursts of enthusiasm and want to get fit as quickly as possible, so they exercise hard and long until they are sore all over. This is not only undesirable, it could even be dangerous. If you are about to take up an energetic sport which you abandoned years ago, make sure you build up your strength first (see page 174), concentrating on the areas which are most likely to be strained by your chosen exercise. Go slowly at first and gradually build up over a period of weeks or even months, until you reach your target level. Start off by doing only half the amount you think you are capable of and don't compare yourself with others. Always start with some gentle warm-up exercises (see page 176) and take at least five minutes to cool down afterwards.

If you know that you have high blood pressure, angina or other heart trouble, consult your doctor about your proposed activity *before* embarking on it. If you have a minor, temporary illness, such as a cold or influenza, it is best not to exercise until you have recovered. If in doubt, always consult your doctor.

SUPPLENESS

You need to develop the maximum range of movement of your joints, back and neck, without causing any strain to your muscles, ligaments or tendons. The more mobile you are, the less likely you are to develop any aches and pains. Stretch exercises increase your flexibility. It is always important to relax the muscles that you are trying to stretch in order to encourage your maximum stretch and prevent injury.

A stretch can be divided into stages:

Total stretch

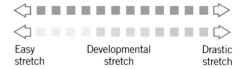

| Easy stretch | Developmental stretch | Drastic stretch |

An easy stretch can be accomplished comfortably when you are completely relaxed. A developmental stretch causes some discomfort and increases with practice. And a drastic stretch is painful and should not be attempted in case it causes injury.

How supple are you?

To test your current suppleness, sit on the floor with your legs stretched out straight in front of you and try to touch your toes. If you can reach them easily, you are very supple; if you can only reach your ankles, you are quite supple and should work on improving your suppleness; and if you can only reach somewhere between your knees and your ankles, you are not very supple.

Swimming, gymnastics, judo and dancing are all good forms of exercise for increasing suppleness, as is yoga, which improves the flexibility of almost every part of the human body.

STAMINA

This means staying power, endurance, or the ability to keep going without gasping for breath. The greater your stamina, the better your circulation, so that plenty of vital oxygen is pumped into working muscles. Stamina is also described as aerobic fitness (see page 178) because it ensures that the oxygen you breathe is used as efficiently as possible. People with greater stamina have a slower, more powerful heartbeat and can cope with more prolonged and strenuous exertion than those with poor stamina. In order to acquire stamina, you must exercise vigorously, for 15-20 minutes three or four times a week.

Testing your stamina tests

If you can walk up and down two flights of stairs (about 20 steps each flight) fairly briskly then hold a conversation without getting out of breath, you have good stamina. If you are over 50, you should be able to run on the spot for two minutes; if you are under 50, you should be able to run for three minutes.

Pulse rate indicates stamina

Your pulse rate is another indication of stamina. It is very easy to learn how to take it (see below). The maximum rate at which a heart can beat is 220 beats per minute, but that rate decreases by one beat for every year of life. To find

out your *maximum* pulse rate, subtract your age from 220. Your pulse rate during exercise – your training pulse rate – *should be 70 per cent of the maximum rate for your age*.

The recommended training pulse rate can also be calculated by subtracting your age from 200, and then subtracting further a handicap of 40 for unfitness (this handicap may be reduced to 20 once you get fitter). For example, if you are 52 and unfit, your training pulse rate should be $200 - 52 = 148 - 40 = 108$.

To begin with you can achieve this by running on the spot. Start by doing this gently for thirty seconds, letting your arms hang down by your side and without attempting to lift your knees too high. Gradually build up to five or six minutes, taking your pulse frequently; do not exceed your prescribed rate.

TAKING YOUR OWN PULSE

The pulse is the wave of pressure that passes along every artery following a heart beat (see page 19). The best way to take your own pulse is to take the pulse in the radial artery at the wrist. Hold one hand palm upwards and place the pads of three fingers of the other hand on the groove on the outer side of the wrist — just below the creases — in line with your thumb. You will be able to feel a pulse quite clearly when your fingers are in the right place.

Use a watch with a second hand. Count the number of beats you can feel in 15 seconds and multiply by four to obtain the rate per minute.

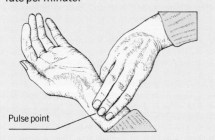

Pulse point

TRAINING PULSE RATES

This chart gives you the recommended range of training pulse rates for various ages up to the age of 60; if you are over 60, you should ask your doctor for guidance. Just as there is a lower limit below which the value of exercise falls off sharply, so there is an upper limit beyond which there is no additional benefit. It is important, in any case not to exceed the upper limit of the range for your age, because it would put undue strain on your heart.

Age	Recommended training pulse rate
20	140 – 170
25	135 – 165
30	130 – 160
35	125 – 155
40	120 – 150
45	115 – 145
50	110 – 140
55	105 – 135
60	100 – 130

Warning for coronary patients

If you are unfit, have angina, high blood pressure, or are recovering from a heart attack, your recommended training pulse rate will be lower. This will certainly be the case if you are taking beta-blockers (see page 74), which artificially suppress the pulse rate. As always, take your doctor's advice; he knows which beta-blockers you are taking and if necessary he can arrange for a special exercise test to determine the pulse rate you should aim for.

Using your muscles correctly

Learning to use the large muscle groups simultaneously, such as those in the arms, legs, chest and trunk, will help to increase your stamina. With practice, you will learn to use only the muscles required for the particular activity at hand and to leave the others relaxed and comfortable. If you watch long-distance runners, for example, you will see that while their legs do the running, the rest of their body remains relaxed.

Guidelines for a graded jogging programme are given later (see page 184). Remember too that you should always start with a period of warm-up exercises (see pages 176 to 177).

STRENGTH

The stronger the body, the greater its chances of meeting physical demands without undue strain or injury. Strengthening exercises help you to maintain a well-proportioned body and prepare you for sudden physical demands such as moving furniture. They are also particularly important in preparing you for certain sports, such as skiing.

Although there is always some overlap, it is important to understand that the exercise that increases your aerobic fitness may not necessarily give you strength, and vice versa (see page 178).

STRENGTH TEST

If you wish to test the strength of your shoulder, chest and arm muscles, try this exercise. If you can do ten press-ups, your strength is good; between six and ten press-ups, it is reasonably good; between three and five press-ups, it is average; and only two or less, it is bad.

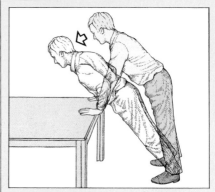

1 Get someone to place a heavy table against a wall and stand 90 to 130 cm (3 to 4ft) away from it with your feet slightly apart. Place both hands on the table.

2 Keeping your body straight, bend your arms so that your chest comes forward to touch the table. Straighten your arms again.

Strength is increased by doing a greater amount of work for a shorter time, such as weight lifting; while stamina is achieved by doing less work for a longer period of time, such as jogging.

SATISFACTION

It is important to enjoy the exercise you do. If you find it boring you won't keep it up, and if you don't practise it regularly you cannot expect any benefits.

It takes 15-20 minutes of vigorous exercise at least three times a week for six weeks before you will notice any significant increase in strength or stamina. The first few sessions may give you nothing more than aching limbs, but,

ACTIVITY SCORES

This table gives you comparative ratings for the suppleness, stamina and strength of various physical activities.

Key	Stamina ◆	Suppleness ●	Strength ■
0 no real effect	**1** beneficial	**2** very beneficial	**3** excellent

Activity	Score ◆	●	■	Activity	Score ◆	●	■
Badminton	1	2	1	Housework (moderate)	0	1	0
Ballet	0	2	1	Hill walking	2	0	1
Basketball	2	2	2	Jogging	3	1	1
Bowling	0	1	1	Judo	1	3	1
Calisthenics	0	1	2	Mowing lawn	1	0	2
Canoeing	2	1	2	Rowing	3	1	3
Climbing stairs	2	0	1	Rugby	2	2	2
Cycling (hard)	3	1	2	Sailing	0	1	1
Dancing (ballroom)	0	2	0	Squash	2	2	1
Dancing (disco)	2	3	0	Swimming (hard)	3	3	3
Digging (garden)	2	1	3	Tennis	1	2	2
Football	2	2	2	Volleyball	0	1	2
Golf	0	1	0	Walking (briskly)	1	0	0
Gymnastics	1	3	2	Weight lifting	0	0	3
Hockey	1	1	1	Yoga	1	3	0

once you get into the habit, you will be sufficiently convinced to want to continue with it, and if you were to give it up your body would undoubtedly miss it. If you practise gentle yoga, you will feel more supple and be aware of a sense of well-being in a matter of days.

Turn your exercise routine into a social event. Jog with a friend or, if you cannot find a regular companion, join an exercise class or sports club.

Exercise should be both convenient and enjoyable. Lay out exercise clothes by your bedside in readiness for your morning's jog. If you have opted for indoor exercises have an illustrated exercise chart on the wall and put on suitable music while you exercise.

WHICH EXERCISE?

There are many recreational sports and activities for you to choose from. Which one you choose will depend on your inclination, your abilities and disabilities, the health of your heart or your blood pressure, the amount of time you have free, your environment and the facilities available. Whatever you choose, work out a plan that suits you best and try to stick to it. If you are in any doubt about whether you are able to do the exercise, consult your doctor.

WARM-UP EXERCISES

Whatever your chosen form of exercise, it is important to warm up before starting any strenuous activity. This is so that your heart does not have to start working hard suddenly to supply the muscles with the extra oxygen and nutrients needed during exercise, as well as to stretch cold or stiff muscles. These yoga-based warm-up exercises are gentle, yet effective, initial movements which stretch your muscles and generally loosen you up before you start swimming or jogging, for example.

NECK ROLLING

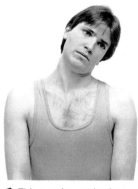

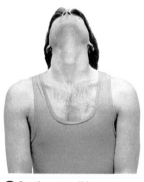

1 This exercise can be done while sitting or standing. Start the exercise by slowly rolling your head round to your left.

2 Continue to roll it round to the back and hold it there briefly. Then slowly roll your head round to the right and hold it there briefly.

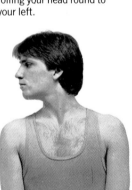

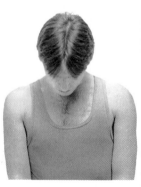

3 Raise your chin and turn your face to the right, as far as is comfortably possible. Then let your chin fall down on to your chest.

4 Gently push your head down as you slowly move it round to the front again. Repeat exercise twice.

SIMPLE FORWARD BENDING

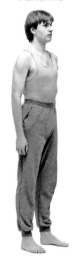

1 Stand upright, with your legs approximately 45cm (18in) apart and your arms by your side. Relax and breathe in.

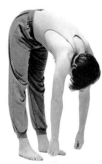

2 Breathe out and bend forwards, letting your arms, head and trunk just hang down as far as possible.

3 Breathing in, straighten up slowly, keeping your arms, hands and head relaxed. Straighten your back first and your head last. Stand upright and breathe out. Repeat 10 times. Increase gradually to 20 times within a week, according to your suppleness.

SIMPLE SIDE BENDING

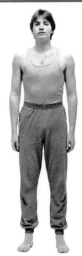
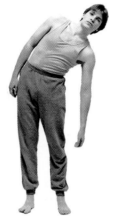

1 Stand upright with your legs approximately 45cm (18in) apart.

2 Breathe in and slowly bend to the left, letting your left hand hang down loosely. Hold for three seconds. Breathe out and slowly straighten up again. Repeat bending to the right. Over about a week, gradually increase the number of repetitions each side from two to ten.

ARM CIRCLING

Stand upright with your feet approximately 45cm (18in) apart. Make a slow circling movement with your arms, breathing in as you raise them and breathing out as you lower them. Repeat ten times. Increase the number to 20 over a week.

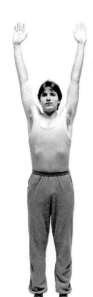
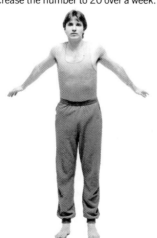

KNEE RAISING

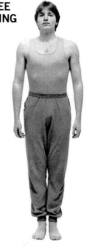

1 Stand with feet together and arms by your sides.

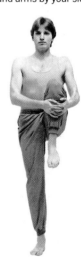

2 Breathe in and gently raise your left knee, grasp your shin and pull it towards your body, keeping your back straight. Hold for three seconds. Breathe out and return to the starting position. Repeat with right leg. Repeat exercise 10 times with each leg, increasing to 20 over a period of a week.

AEROBIC AND ANAEROBIC EXERCISE

Aerobic means, literally, with air, so aerobic exercise is exercise in which the extra energy required is completely fuelled by the extra air you breathe (see page 155). It does not require maximum exertion with each movement but it can be sustained and is carried along by its own, distinctive rhythm. It is the best form of exercise for cardiovascular fitness. Examples of aerobic exercise include walking, jogging, swimming, bicycling, rowing and canoeing.

Anaerobic exercise (without air), on the other hand, consists of brief periods of maximum effort alternated with brief periods of rest and the fuel is not completely burnt. It builds up certain muscles, but it does little for stamina or for the cardiovascular system; it may even put undue strain on it. Examples of anaerobic exercise include raquet and ball games and weight lifting. Do not practise these types of exercise without consulting your doctor.

SWIMMING

This is one of the best forms of exercise you can take. It offers the maximum benefits in terms of stamina, suppleness and strength. High blood pressure, angina, asthma or arthritis are no contra-indication to swimming, provided that you keep within your limits and the water is warm. All these conditions are likely to be helped by swimming. It can also be enjoyed at any age.

If you can't swim, it is well worth learning. Go to your local public baths, where you will probably find that there are special classes which you can join. Alternatively, contact your local authority recreational department or adult education institute for information on swimming lessons.

If you are only an occasional or summer holiday swimmer, build up your swimming schedule gradually. A vigorous 20-minute swim at least three times a week is what you should aim for. Many public pools are open early in the morning at least a couple of times a week, so you can fit in a swim before going to work. If not, try after work but before your evening meal.

Concentrate on a good stretch and streamlined body positions. Remember to breathe freely while you are swimming, as this helps you to relax and swim smoothly. Try a variety of strokes – breast stroke, back stroke, crawl and so on – to exercise different groups of muscles. If you swim in an outdoor pool, make sure that the water is warm and, if you are swimming in the sea or a river, that there are no dangerous currents or tides.

YOGA

I am personally biased in favour of yoga because it is safe at all ages, it is non-competitive, requires no equipment and can be practised in all weathers (indoors or out). It produces an excellent degree of suppleness and, to a lesser extent, stamina and a little strength. It is particularly beneficial for coronary heart disease because it promotes relaxation, thereby helping you to cope with stress, reducing high blood pressure and increasing cardiovascular efficiency.

What is yoga?

Yoga is an ancient Indian philosophy which encompasses the whole man – his spiritual, mental and physical needs. The word yoga is in fact derived from the Sanskrit root "yuj" meaning union, which refers to its purpose of uniting man's physical and spiritual existence. It teaches relaxation, breath control, physical postures, mental exercise and meditation, which together stretch the body, strengthen the mind and enhance spiritual growth.

There are several methods of yoga comprising a series of well thought-out postures, or positions, which exercise virtually every part of the human body. In this chapter I describe some simple yoga exercises; breathing, deep relaxation and meditation are all discussed in detail in Chapter 13, Coping with Stress.

General rules for yoga

● Practise whenever you have time and space, preferably somewhere quiet so that you will not be disturbed.

● Practise half an hour after liquid intake, such as orange juice, one and a half to two hours after a light meal, or three to four hours after a heavy meal.

● Make sure that the room is warm so that you will not be uncomfortable. It should also be well ventilated.

● Always do yogic postures slowly and smoothly. It is better to spend ten minutes doing one posture correctly than four or five postures badly.

● Wear a comfortable, loose-fitting garment such as a track suit.

● Never be tempted to compare your performance with that of others around you. Yoga exercises are non-competitive and every individual is different. Keep within your own comfortable limits by learning to listen to your own body's signals. If a considerable time has elapsed since you stopped exercising,

begin again with no more than 15 minutes to start with and build up over a few weeks.

● Concentrate your mind completely on the posture you are doing. This not only prevents any straining of muscles, joints and ligaments but also makes you aware of the particular part of the body you are moving. This clears the mind of all other thoughts and brings about a profound feeling of relaxation.

● Breathe through your nose slowly and deeply in relationship with the movements. Try to follow the instructions correctly, but if at first you find that you cannot hold your breath for the required count, do not worry – with practice you will be able to hold your breath for longer and longer. If you run out of breath too soon, simply take another one.

● Floor surfaces vary a great deal. For consistency, use the same practice mat wherever you are doing your exercises.

● Yoga is very enjoyable, but it should nevertheless be taken seriously if you are to obtain the maximum benefit.

● Do not exercise if you are ill, for example, if you have a cold or 'flu, wait until you feel better and are strong enough again. Some people believe that women should not exercise during their menstrual periods but should do only deep breathing and, if possible, take short walks.

● Although yoga does improve your health and is useful in eliminating many ailments, it must not be used as a substitute for medical treatment. If in doubt, check with your doctor.

● Always start with warm-up exercises (see page 176) and end with a relaxation posture (see page 161).

● Buy yourself a book on yoga and follow the instructions faithfully or, better still, join a class run by a qualified yoga teacher.

YOGA EXERCISES

I have included some basic yoga exercises for you to try. They are designed to be carried out in a sequence. Each one is divided into stages, so that you can progress as you become more flexible. It will probably take about two weeks to master the first stage. However, do not worry if it takes you more than a fortnight to proceed to the next stage.

CHEST EXPANSION

This exercise is good for "opening up the chest", making it easier for your lungs to expand as you breathe, so that you take in more air with each breath and breathe more efficiently (see page 159). Practise the basic exercise, then, as you become more supple, try the advanced stages.

Stage One

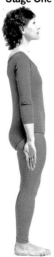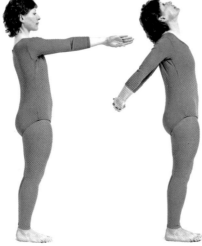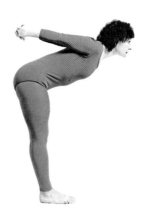

1 Stand up straight in a relaxed posture with your knees together and your arms by your sides, with your palms facing outwards.

2 Bring your hands up to touch your chest, then straighten your arms out. Keeping your arms at shoulder level, bring your arms round behind you.

3 Lower your arms and lock your fingers together. Slowly bend backwards, keeping your arms away from your body and looking upwards.

4 Then, slowly and gently, bend forwards; bring your arms up as high as you can. Relax your neck and look towards your knees. Return to the upright position.

Stage Two (not illustrated)

1 Repeat the exercise as above but bend slightly further backwards and hold the position for ten seconds.

2 Then bend slightly further forwards and hold for ten seconds.

Stage Three

1 Bend as far back as you can and hold this position for five seconds.

2 Then bend as far forwards as you can letting your arms come up as high as possible and try to touch alternate knees with your nose. Hold for 20 seconds then return to the upright position, see right.

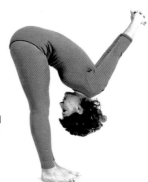

SIMPLE TWIST

This is an excellent exercise for helping to trim your waistline as well as increase cardiovascular efficiency. Begin with stage one. After two weeks of regular practice, try stage two.

Stage One

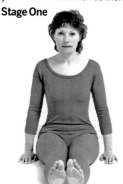 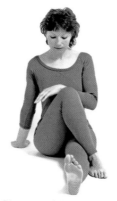 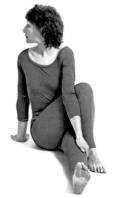

1 Sit on the floor with your legs out in front of you. Breathe in and bend your right leg up and cross it over your left, so that your right foot is level with your knee.

2 Place your right hand behind you. Bring your left hand over your right knee to hold your left knee. Twist as far to the right as possible and hold for five seconds.

3 Breathe out and straighten up again, uncross your legs and extend them in front of you. Repeat the movement twisting to the left.

Stage Two

1 Sit on the floor with your legs extended. Breathe in and bend your knee so that the sole of your left foot is against your right thigh.

2 Bend your right leg up and, holding your ankle with both hands, swing your right leg over your left knee and rest the foot on the floor.

3 Place your right hand flat on the floor behind you and hold your left knee firmly with the other hand.

4 Twist round to the right until you can reach your left side at the waist with your right hand. Hold for ten seconds. Breathe out, release your right hand, and straighten your body. Breathe in, repeat the twist, holding for ten seconds.

5 Slowly straighten up and relax for a minute. Repeat the exercise, turning to the left. Relax for one minute before doing your next exercise.

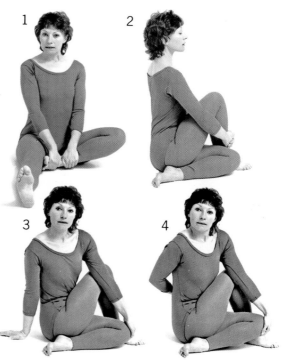

LEG RAISING

This exercise strengthens the muscles in your abdomen; improves blood circulation in the upper body; and relaxes the legs, draining blood back to the heart which can be particularly beneficial if you have varicose veins. The third stage is sometimes known as a shoulder stand.

Stage One

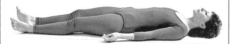

1 Lie down on your back with your hands by your sides. Let your body relax completely.

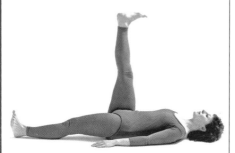

2 Turn your hands palms downwards. Breathe in and slowly raise your right leg up until it is at a right angle to your body. Hold this position for five seconds.

3 Breathe out and gradually lower your leg while you do so. Repeat the exercise with your left leg. Repeat the whole exercise twice more. Gradually build up doing two additional cycles every day until you reach 20 per day. Then move on to stage 2.

Stage Two

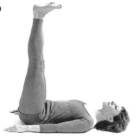

Start as above but this time raise both legs, keeping your feet and knees together all the time. Start with two repetitions and build up gradually until you can do 20.

Stage Three

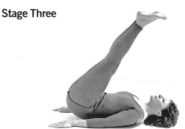

1 Start as before, lying flat on the ground, and raise both legs slowly while pushing down with the palms of your hands. Take your legs forwards over your head, until you can feel your back and hips coming up off the floor.

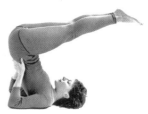

2 Bring both hands up and place them on your waist or lower back, see above. Bring your body up as far as you can and then straighten up — your chin should almost touch your chest, and your abdomen and legs should be in a straight line, see right. Hold this position for a few seconds.

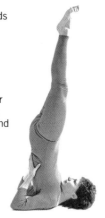

3 It is only possible to reach this position after a great deal of practice so just go as far as you can each time. When you can hold this position for two to five minutes, close your eyes and practise slow, rhythmic breathing while your body is vertical.

COBRA

This is a particularly good exercise for removing all tension, particularly from the back. It also strengthens the abdominal and back muscles and helps you become more supple. Master the basic positions of stages one and two, then move on to the more complicated stage three.

Stage One

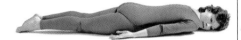

1 Lie on your stomach with your head turned to one side and your arms by your sides. Let your body relax completely.

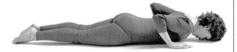

2 Carefully turn your head so that your forehead is touching the floor and place your hands, palms downwards, directly under your shoulders, with your fingers together.

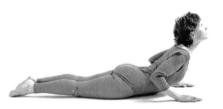

3 As you breathe in, slowly tilt your head backwards, push your hands against the floor, and – gradually – raise your trunk. Hold for five to ten seconds, depending on how comfortable you feel.

4 As you breathe out, bring your head forward and lower your trunk to the floor again. Relax. Repeat the exercise two or three times, gradually increasing the number to ten over a period of about two weeks.

Stage Two (not illustrated)

Do the exercise, as above, but aim to raise the trunk a little further and hold the position for 15 seconds. Repeat two or three times initially and gradually build up to ten.

Stage Three

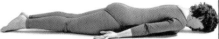

1 Lie down on your stomach with your hands by your sides and relax. Turn your head so that your forehead is touching the floor.

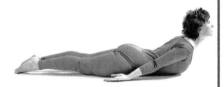

2 Leaving your hands down by your sides, breathe in and raise your head and trunk up off the floor without the support of your hands.

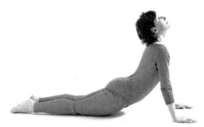

3 Then slowly bring your hands forward, one by one, continuing to raise your trunk. With practice, your head will go back further and further, enabling your elbows to straighten, your abdomen to be raised and back arched while your legs are relaxed. Initially, hold the position for five seconds, gradually increasing it to 15 seconds.

4 Slowly lower your trunk and head, returning your arms to your sides. Gently lower your forehead to the floor. Turn your head to one side and relax.

JOGGING

A dynamic form of exercise, jogging is one of the best exercises for attaining cardiovascular fitness. It requires no equipment except a pair of special running shoes to protect your feet and cushion your entire body against the jarring effect of repeated impact. You should lower your heels first, rocking forwards on them as when you walk. Don't run on your toes.

Jogging should not be competitive. Just run at a pace that makes you mildly breathless. The steady, easy rhythm helps to ease away tension and leaves

JOGGING SCHEDULES

1: Use this programme if you are fairly fit and under 35

Week	Activity
1	Half an hour's brisk walking every day. Walk at every opportunity.
2	Walk 5 mins; jog 30 secs, walk 30 secs repeat x 10; jog 45 secs, walk 45 secs repeat x 3; walk 5 mins.
3	Walk 5 mins; jog 1 min, walk 1 min repeat x 5; walk 5 mins.
4	Walk 2 mins; jog 2 mins, walk 1 min repeat x 10; walk 2 mins.
5 and after	Walk 1 min; jog 3 mins, walk 1 min repeat x 5. Increase jogging time and cut walking breaks until jogging 20 minutes.

2: Use this programme if you are unfit and over 35

Week	Activity
1	Half an hour's brisk walking every day. Walk at every opportunity.
2	Walk 5 mins; jog 15 secs, walk 15 secs repeat x 5; walk 5 mins; jog 15 secs, walk 15 secs repeat x 5; walk 5 mins.
3	Walk 5 mins; jog 30 secs, walk 30 secs repeat x 3; walk 4 mins; jog 30 secs, walk 30 secs repeat x 3; walk 5 mins.
4	Walk 5 mins; jog 1 min, walk 1 min repeat x 2; walk 2 mins; jog 1 min, walk 1 min repeat x 2; walk 5 mins.
5	Walk 5 mins; jog 1 min, walk 1 min repeat x 5; walk 5 mins.
6	Walk 2 mins; jog 2 mins, walk 1 min repeat x 5; walk 5 mins.
7-8	Increase jogging time and cut down walking breaks until jogging 10-20 mins without break.

you feeling refreshed and revitalized. However, if you have high blood pressure, any heart or circulatory disorder or arthritis in your legs, do consult your doctor before you start.

Ideally, you should jog every day. If this is not possible, you must jog on alternate days, otherwise you will lose the training effect. If, however, you are not used to it, you should not just rush out one day and start jogging without preparing yourself first. Begin with brisk walks interspersed with brief jogs.

How long you can jog for depends on your age and your state of fitness. The most important thing is to build up your schedule gradually, week by week, allowing heart, lungs and circulation time to develop stamina. The table opposite gives two programmes which give you an idea of how you should build up your own schedule.

When not to jog

Avoid jogging immediately after a meal or if you are tired or unwell. Many people find that the best time is early in the morning before breakfast, or after work before supper. If you jog in the dark, wear a reflective jacket or light-coloured clothing so that you can easily be seen by motorists. Wear loose-fitting, lightweight clothes that keep you warm, but do not make you too hot.

CAUTION

■ Consult your doctor if you have high blood pressure, any heart condition, a chest complaint like asthma or bronchitis, arthritis, back pain or any other problem which you think could be affected if you go jogging.

■ Beware of rough ground which could cause injury, and if possible, avoid jogging on hard surfaces, such as roads or pavements, since this jars your spine and other joints. Do not jog up and down hills, as this also has a jarring effect.

■ Stop jogging immediately if you feel any chest discomfort.

■ Always wear special running shoes. They should have thick soles with good arch support and heel support. A careless choice of shoes may not only cause discomfort to your feet, but actual injury to your knees and ankles. Avoid those with a plastic lining or high tabs at the back. A good sports shop will be able to advise you.

■ Wear comfortable, loose-fitting clothes and avoid synthetic fabrics in which you could get hot and sweaty. Wear a top that can easily be removed once you have warmed up. Wear light coloured or reflective clothing if you jog in the dark.

■ Do not jog if you are suffering from any temporary illness, however minor, until you have recovered.

■ Do not jog if you feel very tired.

■ Watch out for icy roads in winter and avoid jogging if it is foggy.

CYCLING

This is not only a cheap and enjoyable form of transport, it is also a superb way of keeping fit. It is excellent for building cardiovascular stamina, while at the same time developing good strength and suppleness in your legs. In order to build up adequate stamina, however, you have to push yourself hard for a reasonable period of time – say, about 20 minutes, at least three times a week. Cycling exercises only the large muscles in the legs and is therefore somewhat limited in benefit to other parts of the body. However, as always if you are suffering from high blood pressure or circulatory disorder, do consult your doctor before you start. Buy a bicycle with gears, to help on the hills.

CYCLING PRECAUTIONS

■ Always wear light or reflective clothes so you are visible to motorists. Keep your lights in good working order.

■ Beware of drivers who seem to come from nowhere. Keep well to the inside of the road and, if you are cycling with a friend, remember to stay in single file.

■ Cycling in heavy traffic may mean that you are breathing polluted air, while loud traffic noise can be stressful.

■ Rough road surfaces may lead to discomfort or even injury. Avoid unfamiliar roads in the dark.

■ If you are elderly, stiff or have any form of disability, such as arthritis, avoid cycling in heavy city traffic where co-ordination and swift reflexes are essential for your safety.

■ Always remember to keep your bike locked when it is left anywhere, even outside your own home.

EXERCISE FOR CORONARY PATIENTS

It is very important to build up your cardiovascular efficiency. If you are suffering from angina or coronary heart disease, or recovering from a heart attack, you will probably be advised to attend a coronary rehabilitation centre, where you will probably be given an exercise programme to follow. If you want to join a keep fit or yoga class, make detailed enquiries to ensure that the teacher is qualified to deal with cardiac patients. If you are in any doubt, you must discuss your specific needs with your doctor. Angina sufferers should follow the same guidelines.

Rehabilitation programme

If you go to a coronary rehabilitation centre, you will probably have three exercise sessions per week, each lasting 15 to 20 minutes. Al Murray, British National and Olympic coaching adviser and remedial gymnast, has developed a special series of exercises used in some rehabilitation clinics.

If the centre uses a system based on Al Murray's programme, you will probably start with mobility exercises, such as arm swinging, side bends, trunk, knee and hip bends, head, arm and trunk rotating, and alternate ankle

reaches. Performed slowly while breathing freely, mobility exercises warm you up and make your joints more flexible. Next you will be asked to do various strengthening exercises, such as progressive press ups and abdominal and leg exercises, which aim to condition your muscles and make them more resistant to sudden strain.

Finally you will be asked to do heart and lung exercises such as running on the spot or stepping on and off a bench. The aim of these exercises is to build up the efficiency of your heart gradually in order that you can maintain a prescribed pulse rate for up to 10 minutes (see page 173).

The benefits of a rehabilitation programme based on Al Murray's exercises can be derived from several different forms of exercise that also improve mobility, strength and heart and lung efficiency. The yoga-based warm-up exercises (see page 176) add to mobility, while also helping steady, regular breathing. Swimming (see page 178) also improves all three aspects of fitness, suppleness, strength and stamina, and could be incorporated into a rehabilitation programme, particularly if your return to fitness is progressing well.

Useful addresses

There are many organizations which can supply information about heart disease, offer advice and support, or send you a list of qualified therapists practising in your area. Many of them have a network of branches throughout the country, and if you cannot find your local branch in the telephone directory, the head office listed below can probably give you the address of a branch near you, or put you in touch with somebody who will be able to help you.

GENERAL HEALTH

Health Education Council
78 New Oxford Street
London WC1A 1AH
01-637 1881
(general information service, publishes leaflets)

Scottish Health Education Group
Woodburn House
Canaan Lane
Edinburgh EG10 4SG
031-447 8044
(publishes information leaflets)

Age Concern
Bernard Sunley House
60 Pitcairn Road
Mitcham
Surrey
01-640 5431
(national centre for 950 independent groups serving the needs of elderly people)

HEART DISEASE

British Heart Foundation
102 Gloucester Place
London W1H 4DH
01-935 0185
(publishes information on all aspects of heart disease)

Chest, Heart and Stroke Association
Tavistock Square
London WC1H 9JE
01-387 3012
(publishes information leaflets, offers advice and practical support)

Cardiac Spare Parts Club
10 Duke Street
Little Common
Bexhill-on-Sea
East Sussex

DIABETES

British Diabetic Association
10 Queen Anne Street
London W1
01-323 1531
(publishes information leaflets, has a counselling service and gives practical help)

NUTRITION

The British Nutrition Foundation
15 Belgrave Square
London SW1X 8PS
01-235 4904
(publishes information on diet and offers advice)

Slimming Magazine Club
9 Kendrick Mews
London SW7 3HG
01-225 1711
(for access to a network of 550 local slimming clubs)

The Advertising Standards Authority
Brook House
Torrington Place
London WC1E 7HN
(for queries about food labelling)

ALCOHOLISM

Alcoholics Anonymous Head Office
11 Redcliffe Gardens
London SW10 9BQ
01-352 9779
(offers advice and support to alcoholics; for a local branch see your telephone directory)

Al-Anon
61 Great Dover Street
London SE1
01-403 0888
(for the families of alcoholics)

Alcohol Concern
3 Grosvenor Crescent
London SW1
01-235 4182
(for access to a network of over 40 local council advice centres)

**Accept Alcoholism
Counselling**
Western Hospital
200 Seagrave Road
London SW6
01-381 3155
*(for advice, information and
counselling on alcoholism)*

SMOKING

**Action on Smoking and
Health (ASH)**
5-11 Mortimer Street
London W1
01-637 9843
*(publishes information leaflets
and advice on how to give up)*

EMOTIONAL HELP

Samaritans
39 Walbrook
London EC4
01-283 3400/626 9000
*(24 hour advice service to
anyone in distress)*

*For your local branch, look in
your telephone directory,
either on the emergency
numbers page inside the front
cover, or in the alphabetical
listing.*

KEEPING FIT

Sports Council (England)
16 Upper Woburn Place
London WC1H 0QP
01-388 1277

Sports Council for Wales
National Sports Centre
Sophia Gardens
Cardiff CF1 9SW
0222 397571

Scottish Sports Council
1 St. Colme Street
Edinburgh
031-225 8411
*(Sports Councils have lists of
sports centres in England,
Wales and Scotland and
publish brochures of courses)*

Al Murray
City Gym
Moore Lane
London EC2Y 9BU
01-628 0786
*(runs rehabilitation courses for
heart patients)*

COMPLEMENTARY MEDICINE

**British Holistic Medical
Association**
179 Gloucester Place
London NW1
01-262 5299
(publishes information)

**Institute for
Complementary Medicine**
21 Portland Place
London W1N 3AS
01-636 9543
*(publishes information about
therapies available)*

British Wheel of Yoga
General Secretary
Grafton Grange, Grafton
York YO5 9QQ
090 12 3386
*(provides a list of all qualified
yoga teachers in the UK)*

Massage Techniques
Clare Maxwell-Hudson
87 Dartmouth Road
London NW2 4ER
01-450 6494
*(for information on massage
courses)*

**National Register of
Hypnotherapists and
Psychotherapists**
National College of Hypno-
tists and Psychotherapists
25 Market Square
Nelson, Lancs
0282 699378
*(can supply a list of qualified
practitioners)*

**Centre for Autogenic
Training**
Positive Health Centre
101 Harley Street
London W1
01-935 1811
*(offers group and individual
training)*

Council for Acupuncture
10 Belgrave Square
London SW1X 8PH
*(publishes a list of all British
acupuncturists registered with
three main acupuncture
organizations)*

**St. John's Ambulance
Association**
1 Grosvenor Crescent
London SW1X 7EF
01-235 5231
*(voluntary organization which
runs first aid courses)*

**St. Andrew's Ambulance
Association**
St Andrew's House
Milton Street
Glasgow G4 0HR
041-332 4031
*(voluntary organization which
runs first aid courses)*

British Red Cross Society
9 Grosvenor Crescent
London SW1X 7EJ
01-235 5454
*(voluntary organization which
runs first aid courses)*

Index

ACKNOWLEDGMENTS

Dorling Kindersley would like to thank: Anne Johnson and Claire Le Bas for their editorial help; Diana Burns for proof-reading; Hilary Bird for the index; Jean Coombes and Tim Hammond for modelling the exercises; Dr Peter Nixon and the staff of the Cardiac Department, Charing Cross Hospital; and Anne Crowther, Chief cardiac technician, Mayday Hospital for allowing us to take reference photographs; Al Murray for advice on exercise for heart patients; and Margaret Wyatt for typing the original manuscript.

Illustrators
Nick Hall and Barbara Hyams
Photographer
Paul Fletcher
Additional illustrations and chart sources
☐ p.36 Department of Medical Illustration, St. Bartholomew's Hospital, London
☐ p.39 Table taken from John R. Hampton, Cardiovascular disease, Heinemann, London
☐ p.40 Graph: Professor Michael Marmot,

Post-graduate medical journal, Jan 1984
☐ pp. 42, 44, 45 Graphs produced from figures taken from the Framingham Study Mass. USA
☐ p.53 Stress test: Western center for Preventive and Behavioural Medicine Inc. Stress Management series
☐ p.55 Behaviour test: W. Bortner, Journal of Chronic diseases 1969, 22: 87-91
☐ p.59 Stress test: T.H. Holmes and R.H. Rahe, Journal of Psychosomatic Research 1967, 2: 213
☐ p. 138 and 184: charts reproduced by kind permission of the Health Education Council, London
☐ p. 145 smoker test: Merseyside Cancer Education Committee

Typesetting
Rowland Phototypesetting (London) Ltd
Reproduction
Reprocolor Llovet Barcelona SA